Dermatology

pocket tutor

Dermatology

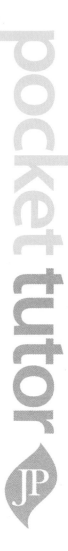

Emma Craythorne MBChB MRCP
Consultant Dermatologist and
Dermatological Surgeon
Dermatology Surgery and Laser Unit
St John's Institute of Dermatology
St Thomas' Hospital
London, UK

Marie-Louise Daly MB BChir MPhil (Cantab)
MRCP Derm
Specialist Registrar in Dermatology
St John's Institute of Dermatology
St Thomas' Hospital and King's College Hospital
London, UK

JP
medical
publishers

© 2015 JP Medical Ltd.

Published by JP Medical Ltd, 83 Victoria Street, London, SW1H 0HW, UK

Tel: +44 (0)20 3170 8910   Fax: +44 (0)20 3008 6180

Email: info@jpmedpub.com   Web: www.jpmedpub.com

ISBN: 978-1-907816-78-9

British Library Cataloguing in Publication Data
A catalogue record for this book is available from the British Library

Library of Congress Cataloging in Publication Data
A catalog record for this book is available from the Library of Congress

Publisher:	Richard Furn
Development Editor:	Thomas Fletcher
Editorial Assistant:	Katie Pattullo
Design:	Designers Collective Ltd

Typeset, printed and bound in India.

Preface

All doctors, regardless of specialty, will encounter patients with skin disease. This book provides a concise guide to the investigation, diagnosis and management of common skin diseases.

The first four chapters give an understanding of the structure and function of the skin and the processes required to make a dermatological diagnosis. Subsequent chapters are arranged by disease type and summarise the clinical features and management options for each diagnosis, alongside diagrams and photographs to aid understanding. Finally, there are chapters covering dermatological emergencies and the principles of dermatological surgery.

We hope that this book will benefit both students and trainee doctors, by acting as a quick reference to use in the clinic and in preparation for exams.

Emma Craythorne
Marie-Louise Daly
March 2015

Contents

Acknowledgements

A huge thank you to our dermatology trainees, particularly Bryan Macdonald and Karolina Gholam, and to my colleagues at the St John's Institute of Dermatology. Thanks to Tanya Henshaw for her contribution to the nursing chapter and also to Rhonda Meys. Thanks to Gary Mulcahy for the medical photography, and a special thanks to Anthony du Vivier, a mentor and friend who is responsible for making this book happen. Finally, thanks to my husband Neil, who now knows more dermatology than he ever thought possible.

EC

I would like to thank David McGibbon for his help with supplying images, my great friends and colleagues Bláithín Moriarty and Seshi Manam for their help, and Rachael Morris-Jones, David and Elaine for their good humour and advice. Final and most special thanks go to Philippa for her unwavering support and encouragement.

M-LD

First principles

The skin is a remarkable structure upon which we are completely dependent to protect the internal organs from the external environment. Dermatology is the study of all the skin and its adnexal structures.

- Skin disease is common, accounting for 25% of patient visits to a family doctor
- There are more than 2000 specific skin diseases, and many more subtypes are known
- Skin disease is not commonly associated with mortality, but there is a high association with morbidity
- Skin disease can have serious psychosocial effects
- Skin lesions may be the presenting feature of an underlying systemic illness

Sound knowledge of the normal function and anatomy of the skin enables us to understand how symptoms and physical signs relate to disease. The clinical signs seen in the skin are a consequence of the underlying pathological process, so being able to interpret what you see will lead to the diagnosis.

1.1 Functions of the skin

The anatomy of the skin reflects the many functions that it has to perform; at certain sites the skin is anatomically subtly different to allow for a specific role. In general the skin allows for a stable internal environment because it:

- acts as a physical and immunological barrier, protecting the body from chemical, antimicrobial, heat and radiation damage
- regulates body temperature by evaporation of sweat in warm weather and constricting blood vessels and contracting arrector pili (goose bumps) muscles in cold weather
- maintains fluid balance by excreting water and salts (sweat) and preventing water loss from the body due to close contact of keratinocytes in the epidermis

In addition, the skin:

- facilitates awareness of temperature, pain, touch and vibration
- acts as a means of communication in terms of our appearance, odour (apocrine gland secretion) and skin colour
- is responsible for synthesis of vitamin D and storage of fat in the subcutaneous tissue
- forms nails, which protect the digits, enable scratching and add to dexterity

1.2 The biology of normal skin

The skin is the largest organ in the body and is composed of three layers, each contributing to the special functions of the skin (**Figure 1.1**):

1. epidermis
2. dermis
3. subcutis

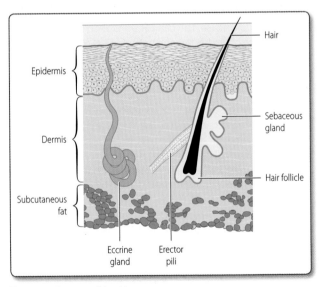

Figure 1.1 Structure of the skin.

Epidermis

The epidermis (**Figure 1.2**) is the outermost part of the skin and is in a constant state of regeneration. The thickness of this layer is site-specific and can range from 0.03 mm on the eyelids to 1.5 mm on the soles of the feet.

The main cell types of the epidermis are:

- keratinocytes
- melanocytes
- Langerhans' cells
- Merkel's cells

Keratinocytes

These are organised into layers, based on distinct structural features. The basal layer consists of a single layer of keratinocytes, which are the active stem cells. These cells proliferate and commit daughter cells to terminal differentiation as they move to the skin surface. The average transit time for a cell to travel from the stratum germinativum to the stratum corneum is 40–56 days. The 'brick wall' structure of the epidermis is provided by desmosomes, which hold the cells together.

The distinct layers of the epidermis (**Figure 1.2**) are as follows.

Stratum germinativum (basal cell layer) This is composed of columnar epithelium cells arranged on their short axis. The cells

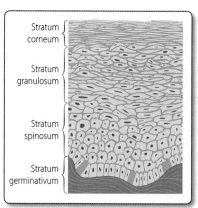

Stratum corneum

Stratum granulosum

Stratum spinosum

Stratum germinativum

Figure 1.2 'Brick wall' structure of the epidermis: the keratinocytes are like the bricks and the lipid mixture surrounding them is like the mortar.

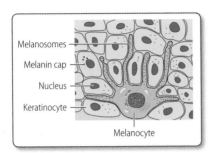

Figure 1.3 Melanocytes synthesise melanin to protect keratinocytes.

Melanosomes

Melanin cap

Nucleus

Keratinocyte

Melanocyte

are the active stem cells, where cell division starts; the cells then undergo terminal differentiation.

Stratum spinosum (prickle layer) Column-shaped keratinocytes move into the stratum spinosum from the stratum basale. They become polygon-shaped and start to synthesise keratin. The spiny appearance of the cells is due to desmosomes.

Stratum granulosum (granular layer) Here the cells have a granular appearance due to keratohyalin granules. Lipids are produced at this layer to form a water barrier. In the transition to the next layer the cells lose their nuclei and organelles.

Stratum corneum This is formed of flattened non-viable corneocytes, usually several layers thick. On the palms and soles this layer is thicker, whereas on mucous membranes it is absent.

Melanocytes (cells producing pigment)

These are dendritic cells derived from the neural crest that are also found in the basal layer at a ratio of 1:10 to basal keratinocytes. Melanocytes synthesise melanin, which is packed into melanosomes and transported to basal keratinocytes (**Figure 1.3**). The melanosomes form a 'melanin cap', which protects the basal keratinocyte from UV-induced DNA damage.

Colour of the skin

This is determined by a number of factors. Fitzpatrick's skin type (**Table 1.1**) is a numerical classification of the colour and the skin's response to UV light. Skin colour is due to the amount of melanin produced by the melanocytes and distributed to the keratinocytes.

Skin type	Characteristics
I	Pale white skin, blue eyes, blonde/red hair Easy to burn, does not tan
II	Fair skin, blue/green eyes, blonde/brown hair Burns easily, tans slightly
III	White skin with golden tone, brown eyes, brown hair Burns and then tans
IV	Light brown skin, brown/black hair Minimal burn, tans easily
V	Brown skin, brown/black hair Rarely will burn and tans dark easily
VI	Black skin, black hair Never burns and tans very easily

Table 1.1 Fitzpatrick's skin types

The most common form of biological melanin is eumelanin, a brown–black polymer derived from the amino acid tyrosine; it is found in the brown colour in skin and hair.

> **Clinical insight**
>
> It is the number and size of the melanosomes, not the number of melanocytes, that determine skin colour.

Pheomelanin, which has a pink-to-red hue, is found in particularly large quantities in red hair, the lips, nipples and glans penis.

Langerhans' cells (antigen-presenting immune cells)

These bone marrow-derived cells have a role in skin immunity: recognition, uptake and presentation of antigens to sensitised T cells. They are dendritic cells found in the mid-epidermis.

Merkel's cells (touch receptors)

These are scarce, small, round cells which transmit sensory information in the skin to the sensory nerves.

> **Clinical insight**
>
> Filaggrin is a protein found in the granular cell layer of the epidermis; its role is to retain water within the keratinocytes. Mutations in filaggrin give rise to dermatoses such as atopic dermatitis. Loss of barrier control, and inflammation and infection, can occur (**Figure 1.4**).

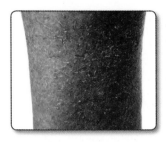

Figure 1.4 Filaggrin mutation note the dry scaling of the skin due to loss of an effective barrier.

Dermoepidermal junction

This is the meeting point of the dermal and epidermal layers of the skin by means of the basement membrane zone (BMZ) (**Figure 1.5**). This zone comprises a network of molecules linking the keratin filaments of the basal keratinocytes to the collagen fibres in the superficial dermis. The main functions of the BMZ are to provide adhesion between the epidermis and the dermis, and to provide a means of communication between cell types.

The basal layer of the epidermis is held and anchored by hemidesmosomes and keratin intermediate filaments. The basal keratinocytes rest on the basal lamina. This serves as a permeable barrier for communication between cells, structural support and a template for wound healing.

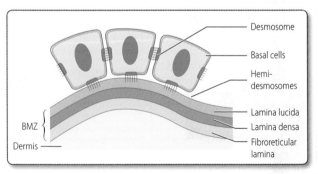

Figure 1.5 Basement membrane zone, with the connecting fibres from the basal keratinocytes to the dermis.

Dermis

The dermis provides the nutrition and support to the epidermis. It is between 1 and 4 mm thick, depending on age and body site. It is divided into two layers: the papillary dermis, which is in contact with the BMZ, and the reticular dermis beneath it. The dermis consists of collagen (90%), elastin fibres (10%) and ground substance (glycoproteins and proteoglycans), and a cellular component of fibroblasts, mast cells, plasma cells and histiocytes. Collagen is a triple-stranded helical molecule, coiled and cross-linked to form microfibrils. The microfibrils are arranged into bundles, which are further organised into collagen fibres. Elastin is generally confined to the lower part of the dermis, where the fibres are arranged in parallel. Blood vessels, lymphatic channels, Meissner's corpuscles (responsible for pressure sensation) and pacinian corpuscles (for sensing vibration) are also found within the dermis.

> ### Clinical insight
>
> Defects in the proteins and glycoproteins at the basement membrane can lead to separation of the dermis and epidermis, with mild trauma and the clinical signs of blistering, as seen in epidermolysis bullosa (**Figure 1.6**).

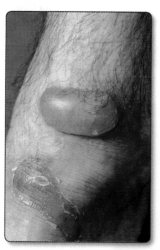

Figure 1.6 Blistering of the skin in a child with epidermolysis bullosa, with separation of the epidermis and dermis.

Fibroblasts

These are the predominant cell type in the dermis; they are responsible for the synthesis and degradation of the connective tissue, and are the key cells in wound healing. **Figure 1.7** shows abnormal overactive wound healing, which can lead to the formation of keloid scars.

Mast cells

These are histamine-containing cells located near dermal blood vessels. They are responsible for immediate-type hypersensitivity reactions.

Glomus bodies

These consist of an arteriovenous shunt surrounded by a capsule of connective tissue. They are found in large numbers in the fingers and toes. Their role is to shunt blood away from the skin surface when exposed to cold temperatures, to prevent heat loss.

Adnexal structures

The pilosebaceous follicles (hair and sebum) and the eccrine (sweat) glands are structures embedded within the dermis, but are derived from and are continuous with the epidermis.

The pilosebaceous unit **(Figure 1.8)** consists of the hair follicle and the sebaceous glands, responsible for the production and secretion of sebum.

- The eccrine glands are not connected to the hair follicle (see Figure 1.1) and open directly on to the skin surface. They

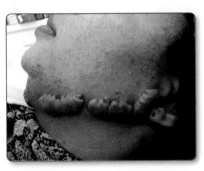

Figure 1.7 Keloid formation secondary to pseudofolliculitis barbae.

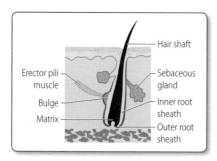

Figure 1.8 Structure of the pilosebaceous unit.

Hair shaft

Erector pili muscle

Bulge

Matrix

Sebaceous gland

Inner root sheath

Outer root sheath

function to regulate body temperature by excreting sweat to allow cooling.

- Apocrine glands are larger than eccrine glands. They release region-specific secretions that bacteria act on and are commonly found in the axilla and genital skin.

Structure of hair

Humans have up to five million hairs over the surface of the skin. Most of this is vellus hair, which is a fine short hair distributed over most of the body. Terminal hair is the longer and coarser hair that is typically found on the scalp, and in the axillae and the pubic area.

The structure of the hair follicle is shown in Figure 1.8. Hair grows from a highly active matrix within the hair bulb, moving along the inner root sheath. Each follicle is made up of three parts: the cortex and medulla, which have pigment cells and are responsible for the colour of the hair, and the cuticle, which is keratinised and provides the strength of the hair.

The hair's course passes the sebaceous gland, and the lipid-rich sebum lubricates it before it exits the skin. The arrector pili muscle inserts into the hair bulb and is responsible for contraction in the cold ('goose bumps'). An important structure within the hair follicle is the hair bulge, where the epithelial and melanocytic stem cell populations reside. This is important in generating hair follicles and sebaceous glands, and re-epithelisation during wound healing (**Figure 1.9**).

Hair growth is a dynamic process with three distinct phases (see **Figure 1.10**):

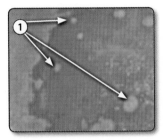

Figure 1.9 A wound bed that is allowed to heal by granulation will show within it islands of re-epithelialisation originating around the hair follicles. ① Island of re-epithelialisation in ulcerated skin.

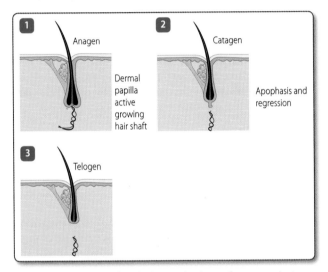

Figure 1.10 The hair growth cycle, showing the changes from anagen (active growing hair), catagen (rest phase of the hair) and telogen (shedding of the hair).

Clinical insight

Keloid formation (**Figure 1.7**) can occur as a consequence of overactive fibroblast activity in response to dermal injury.

1. **Anagen:** hair is actively growing (4–7 years).
2. **Catagen:** hair has stopped growing but cellular activity continues in the hair bulb (several weeks).

3. **Telogen**: there is no growth of hair or any activity in the hair bulb (a few months). This is a resting phase until the cycle is repeated.

As the new anagen hair germinates within the same

> ### Clinical insight
>
> Acne vulgaris, a disorder of the pilosebaceous unit, occurs due to plugging of the hair follicle and sebaceous gland hyperactivity, leading to comedones and inflammatory papules.

follicle, it pushes out the telogen hair. Each hair follicle is independent and goes through the growth phases at different times.

Subcutis

This layer is immediately below the dermis and consists of predominantly adipocytes (fat cells) organised into lobules separated by septa, used mainly for fat storage. It also consists of fibrous bands anchoring the deep fascia, and elastin and collagen fibres attaching it to the dermis. It contains blood vessels, lymphatics and nerves en route to the dermis.

Regional skin variation

Thickness of the epidermis varies; at glabrous sites (non-hair-bearing skin) the stratum corneum is up to 10 times thicker than at non-glabrous sites.

Within non-glabrous skin the hair follicle type and density can vary between different body sites and through different stages of life, e.g. terminal hair follicles may give way to vellus hair follicles in the scalp. In areas such as the axillae, in addition to eccrine glands, apocrine glands are present.

Structure of nail

The nail consists of the nail plate, bed, matrix, proximal and lateral folds, and hyponychium (**Figure 1.11**). The nail matrix is a wedge-shaped structure that contains highly specialised epithelium which produces the cornified cells of the nail plate. The nail plate is visible proximal to the nail fold and grows along the nail bed to the distal free edge of the plate. The nail bed is tightly connected to the nail plate and is continually

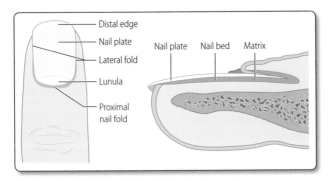

Figure 1.11 Structure of the nail plate.

keratinised to maintain that adhesion. Fingernails grow 0.1 mm/day and toenails 0.03 mm/day.

The nail contributes to tactile sensation and acts as protection for the nail tip. There are glomus bodies in the nail bed and matrix; these are temperature-sensitive organs involved with skin thermoregulation.

1.3 Dermatological terminology

It is essential that the formal language of dermatology is used to describe, record and communicate examination findings accurately (see Chapter 2). A guide to the names of different types of skin lesions is shown in **Table 1.2**.

The underlying pathology correlates well with the physical signs seen in the skin, although it is imperative to take the pathology diagnosis in context with the clinical case, e.g. lichen planus and lichenoid keratosis would be histologically identical, yet the former presents as a widespread rash and the latter as an individual lesion.

Type	Description	Clinical example
Macule	Completely flat lesion, a change in colour (< 1 cm)	Freckle (**Figure 1.12**)
Patch	A large macule	Vitiligo
Papule	Raised lesions < 5 mm; they usually originate in the dermis	Insect bites (**Figure 1.13**)
Nodule	A large raised lesion > 5 mm	Basal cell carcinoma
Plaque	An elevated, broad lesion with a flat surface	Bowen's disease (**Figure 1.14**)
Weal	Elevated lesion from local dermal oedema, with a surrounding flare or border	Urticaria (**Figure 1.15**)
Pustule	A papule containing purulent material, usually of epidermal or upper dermal origin	Acne (**Figure 1.16**)
Abscess	Larger or deeper collections usually in the dermis or subcutis	Abscess
Vesicle	Clear, fluid-filled blisters < 6 mm in diameter	Herpes simplex virus (**Figure 1.17**)
Bullae	Blisters > 6 mm diameter	Bullous pemphigoid
Scale	White accumulation of horny cell layer, implying an epidermal component	Psoriasis (**Figure 1.18**)
Crust	Yellow–brown; consists of dried serum, blood or pus	Impetigo
Erosion	Results from loss of part or all of epidermis	Pemphigus vulgaris (**Figure 1.19**)
Ulcer	Deeper than erosion and includes dermal loss	Leg ulcers
Atrophy	Thinning of the skin with loss of surface marking; visible superficial blood vessels	Excess use of topical corticosteroid
Lichenification	Roughened skin with enhanced skin markings	Chronic eczema, particularly at joint surfaces. Eczema
Hypo-pigmentation	Change in colour of the skin to be lighter	
Hyper-pigmentation	Change in colour of the skin to be darker	Post-inflammatory (**Figure 1.20**)

Table 1.2 A guide to the types of skin lesions

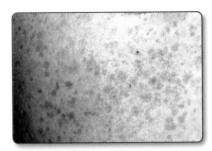

Figure 1.12 Freckles are macular lesions. They are entirely flat and flush with the surrounding skin.

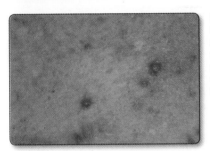

Figure 1.13 Papules are small and palpable. In this example the papules are clustered together on the chest and are itchy; the diagnosis is an insect bite reaction.

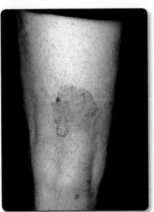

Figure 1.14 A plaque of Bowen's disease. Intraepidermal squamous cell carcinoma is often confused with psoriasis.

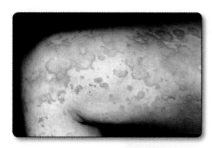

Figure 1.15 Weals of urticaria on the leg.

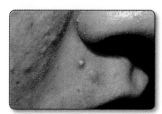

Figure 1.16 Pustule on a background of acneiform skin.

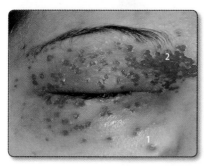

Figure 1.17 This patient has eczema herpeticum. Herpes simplex virus complicating eczema. Note the vesicle [1] and multiple punched out erosions coalescing together [2].

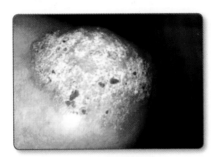

Figure 1.18 Scale is seen overlying an erythematous plaque in psoriasis.

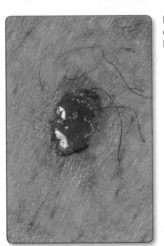

Figure 1.19 Erosion. There is complete loss of the epidermis in this lesion of pemphigus vulgaris.

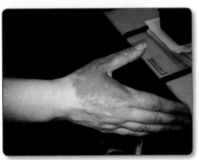

Figure 1.20 Post-inflammatory hyperpigmentation following phytophotodermatitis to lime juice. Note the patient was left handed and used the knife in the left hand and held the lime in the right hand to cut it.

Clinical essentials

For dermatological diagnosis a detailed history, a thorough examination, accurate observations and, sometimes, use of a laboratory are required. Many skin diseases do not have a known cause; a presumptive diagnosis is based on a combination of the signs, symptoms and investigation findings. This chapter details the essential clinical skills that you will need to make a dermatological diagnosis.

2.1 Dermatological history taking

History taking should follow an orderly framework centred on the presenting complaint. This involves a focused systematic approach, as for any other organ system. The process will be quicker for simple benign tumours, but take much longer for identification of the cause of a widespread erythematous eruption.

The 10 key elements of dermatological history taking are described in **Table 2.1**.

History of the presenting complaint

An attempt must be made to elicit answers to the following questions:

- How, where and when did the lesions/rash first present?
- How have the lesions evolved?
- Have there been any previous episodes?
- Are there any symptoms associated with them, e.g. pain, burning or itch?
- Does anything make them better or worse?
- Have you had any previous medications to try to treat them?
- Are there any symptoms on mucosal surfaces, hair-bearing sites or nails?
- What impact has this had on your life?

Systemic enquiry

The systemic enquiry involves the following.

Main heading	Key questions
History of presenting complaint	Nature, site and evolution
	Exacerbating and relieving factors
Systemic enquiry	Fevers, myalgia, arthralgia
Drug history	Over-the-counter, new, old topical medications
Social and environmental history	Occupation and hobbies
	Travel and sun exposure
	Home environment
Family history	Similar problem or other skin disease
Past medical history	Diabetes, sarcoid, autoimmune disease
Psychological history	Anxiety, depression, current stress level
Site-specific history	Nails, genitals, hair
Ideas, concerns, expectations	Related to the skin disease
Summarise	Recap and relate information

Table 2.1 A complete dermatological history

- Are there any generalised systemic features – temperature regulation, myalgia, arthralgia, night sweats? The rash may be part of a systemic problem.
- Any recent illness should be noted because conditions such as erythema multiforme and urticaria may be triggered by viral or bacterial infections, or the drugs used to treat past infections.
- Progress to individual systemic enquiry.

Drug history

For the drug history ask about:

- **medicines taken on or around the onset** of the rash. Ensure that all medications, e.g. vitamins or herbal remedies, are specifically asked about – the condition may be a drug reaction.
- **timing** of the start and end dates of all recent drug prescriptions.
- **any known drug allergies**.

Social and environmental history

For the social and environmental history ask about the following.

- **Occupation(s) and hobbies** – if you suspect a contact or irritant dermatitis, it is important to ask if symptoms improve when away from the particular environment.
- **History of contact** with other affected individuals.
- **Recent travel abroad** – it is important to be aware of endemic diseases in other parts of the world.
- **Recent illness or other stressful events** – certain conditions, e.g. psoriasis, may worsen at times of stress.
- **Anything new in the home environment** or any known allergens – food, pets, furniture, a house move, etc. These may all introduce an allergen that triggers an allergic contact or irritant dermatitis.
- **Sun exposure** history – tanning booths, etc.
- **Smoking habits** – many conditions are related directly to smoking or display a more severe phenotype as a consequence of smoking, such as psoriasis, hidradenitis suppurativa and palmoplantar pustulosis.

Family history

For the family history ask about the following:

- Does anyone in the family have a similar problem?
- Does anyone in the family have a disorder of the skin? Some skin conditions, e.g. neurofibromatosis, have a strong genetic basis; others, e.g. psoriasis or atopic eczema, may have a multifactorial genetic basis but can still help point towards the diagnosis.

Past medical history

This is important because many common systemic diseases display skin manifestations (**Table 2.2**).

Psychological history

People with severe, chronic skin disease may suffer from anxiety, depression and social isolation. Equally the psychological problems may be the cause of the skin disease, e.g. dermatitis artefacta.

Condition	Skin manifestations
Cushing's syndrome	Bruising, striae, acne, hirsutism
Addison's disease	Hyperpigmentation of skin and mucous membranes, hirsutism
Internal malignancy	Dermatomyositis , pemphigus, vasculitis, annular erythemas, Sweet's syndrome, pruritus
Diabetes mellitus	Necrobiosis lipoidica, neuropathic leg ulceration, skin infections
HIV	Maculopapular rash at seroconversion, Kaposi's sarcoma, multiple head-and-neck molluscum contagiosum
Sarcoidosis	Lupus pernio, erythema nodosum
Lupus	Malar rash, photosensitivity, vasculitis
Coeliac disease	Dermatitis herpetiformis

Table 2.2 Skin manifestations of common systemic diseases

Site-specific dermatology history

For some body sites and disease types there are specific details from the history that should be elicited.

Pigmented lesions

History is centred on evolution of the lesion and assessment of the risk factors for skin malignancy (**Table 2.3**).

Scalp

The following factors can affect the scalp:

- **Diet and nutrition**: low serum ferritin (vegetarians) may contribute to telogen effluvium.
- **Menstrual history**: irregular periods may indicate hormonal imbalance.
- **Hair styling history**: physical or chemical methods of treating the hair can lead to damage.
- **Recent stressful events**: dramatic weight loss or illness may lead to a telogen effluvium.

General history	Lesion-specific
Lifelong sun exposure, occupation and hobbies	Changes in shape
Burning episodes	Increase in size
Use of tanning booths	Changes of colour
Family or personal history of skin disease	Changes in the border

Table 2.3 Key factors in the history of a pigmented lesion

Genital
Sexual history: many genital dermatoses result in dyspareunia.

Psychosocial issues
Personal stress may exacerbate many dermatological conditions. It is important to ask about the effect the disease is having on stress levels and also establish if stress may be the cause of the dermatoses.

Ideas, concerns and expectations
It is important to understand what the patient expects the outcome to be. Ask the following.
- What does the patient think may be causing the problem?
- Does the patient have any particular concerns/worries?

Summarise to the patient
It is important to review your findings with the patient; this gives both you and the patient the opportunity to discuss anything and brings a natural end to the history taking.

2.2 Common dermatological symptoms

Key symptom 1: pruritus
This may be localised to one area or be more widespread. It may or may not have skin signs associated with it. Some diseases have a characteristic itch associated with them, which may be helpful in guiding you to a diagnosis, for example:

- widespread itch that is worse at night – atopic dermatitis and systemic reaction (drug, viral, autoimmune)
- intensely pruritic papules – scabies and lichen planus

Key symptom 2: pain

Pain is usually felt as a consequence of a volume effect or due to neural stimulation. Painful lesions include:

- erythema nodosum
- ischaemic ulceration
- cellulitis
- leiomyomas
- angiolipomas

Key symptom 3: evolution

This key symptom enables you to narrow down your differential diagnoses. The patient's description is helpful, for example:

- pain in a dermatomal area before vesicles appear can guide to a diagnosis of in herpes zoster
- pityriasis rosea will start with a herald patch before evolving to a 'Christmas tree pattern' on the back
- presence of a myxoid cyst on the proximal nailfold before nail-plate destruction

2.3 Dermatological physical examination

A thorough dermatological examination includes not only the lesions with which the patient presents but also the entire visible skin, hair, nails and mucous membranes. This is not always appropriate for a readily identifiable disease, but if not performed important findings may be missed. For patients with skin cancer a complete and thorough examination is essential. Documentation is a requirement; the use of a body map can be helpful in documenting complicated conditions (**Figure 2.1**).

Requirements

The following are the requirements for a dermatological examination:

- good lighting

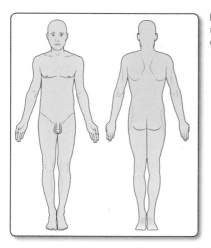

Figure 2.1 Body map used to record examination findings.

- gown for the patient
- chaperone where necessary
- measuring tape, gloves, dermatoscope or magnifying glass, and flashlight

Tip: make it a habit to use the same routine ordered approach to avoid missing important signs.

Systematic skin check

Inspect each part of the body, and do so in the same order each time. Make a note of all abnormal findings:

- **Skin surfaces**: start at the face and continue to the trunk, upper limbs and lower limbs, examining all aspects of the skin. Make a note of palmar plantar lesions.
- **Nails**: examine the nail unit, noting changes to the nail plate, periungal area, cuticles and surrounding skin area.
- **Scalp and hair**: make a note of any areas of hair loss and the hair's texture. Note any changes to the skin of the scalp. Perform a hair-pull test to examine the root if there is hair loss; a lock of hair (approximately 60–80 hairs) is pulled three times (**Figure 2.2**); extraction of two to three hairs is normal, more than six excessive.

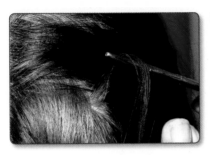

Figure 2.2 Hair-pull test.

- **Mucous membranes**: conjunctivae, visible nasal mucosa, lips, and intraoral and genital areas should be examined where appropriate.

Inspect

General observation is made to determine if the patient is healthy and systemically well, with good body habitus and skin colour. The lesions are identified as a localised or generalised eruption.

Describe

Lesions found should be characterised and the following carefully noted.

- **Distribution**: this will often suggest aetiology, e.g. a systemic process such as viral infection would be more likely to cause a generalised eruption. If the lesions are confined to a single spinal nerve root, a dermatome, this would be a classic scenario for herpes zoster (**Figure 2.3**).
- **Arrangement**: describing the pattern seen can lead to the diagnosis, e.g. a well-demarcated eruption in the same pattern as the contact with a known allergen would suggest a contact dermatitis (**Figure 2.4**).
- **Individual lesions:** the shape, size, colour and surface characteristics should be noted (Table 1.2).

Key sign 1: distribution

Noting the pattern of distribution of eruption in many of the common dermatoses is the key to forming your list of

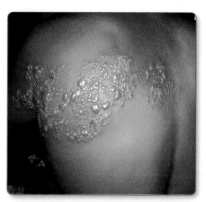

Figure 2.3 Reactivation of herpes zoster 'shingles' presents in a dermatomal distribution.

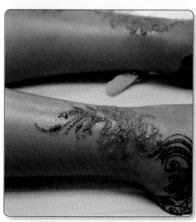

Figure 2.4 Contact dermatitis to *p*-phenylene-diamine in a henna tattoo.

differential diagnoses (**Figure 2.5**). Some conditions will present only on certain body sites, e.g. hair-bearing sites or the flexors, as a consequence of the disease process; other conditions present at certain body sites because of the causative agent.

Many of the common dermatoses have a preference for specific body sites:

- scalp:
    - alopecia areata, androgenic alopecia
    - psoriasis, seborrhoeic dermatitis
    - non-melanoma skin cancers, pilar cysts

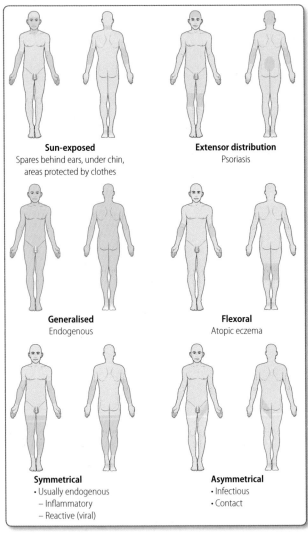

Figure 2.5 The distribution of the lesion points towards the underlying aetiology.

- eyelids:
  - irritant or contact dermatitis, rosacea
  - xanthelasma, apocrine cyst, syringomas, basal cell carcinoma (BCC)
- face:
  - seborrhoeic dermatitis, acne, rosacea
  - impetigo, herpes simplex
  - actinic keratosis, squamous cell carcinoma (SCC), BCC, lentigo maligna
- palmoplantar areas:
  - psoriasis, contact, irritant, atopic dermatitis
  - human papillomavirus (HPV), fungal infection, *Candida* species
- axillae:
  - hidradenitis suppurativa, acanthosis nigricans
  - contact or irritant dermatitis
- genitals:
  - psoriasis, contact or irritant dermatitis
  - lichen planus, lichen sclerosus
  - intraepithelial neoplasia or SCC

Key sign 2: arrangement

The arrangement of the lesions will often create a characteristic pattern that can help to clinch the diagnosis. Lesions may be:

- **clustered**: all in one location, as seen in insect bites, warts, lichen planus
- **satellite**: cluster of lesions around a central area, e.g. metastases in transit
- **confluent**: multiple lesions merging together (**Figure 2.6**)
- **disseminated**: scattered all over the body, e.g. chicken pox
- **erythroderma**: generalised erythema >90%

Key sign 3: individual lesions
Colour

The colour of the background skin should be noted because this may make the colour of dermatoses more difficult to detect. Vitiligo is easier to detect in darker skin types, and erythema easier to detect in lighter skin types. For individual lesions the range of colours is vast, e.g. the colour red is rarely a pure red

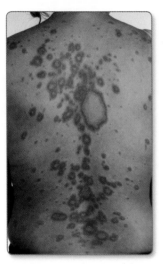

Figure 2.6 Subacute cutaneous lupus: the lesions are merging together.

Clinical insight

Köbner's phenomenon occurs during the active phase of an inflammatory process; new lesions of the inflammatory dermatoses appear within areas of trauma or new scar.

and will often have a hue of orange or purple to it. In addition, the pigmented colour of a naevus may have a number of brown colours within it on close inspection. Drugs can have an impact on and change the colour of the skin (**Table 2.4**).

Shape

Lesional shape is described as follows.

Linear: This type of lesion can occur as a consequence of trauma, developmental or contact allergy, or Köbner's phenomenon.

Annular: These lesions occur as a consequence of circumferential growth of they lesion with central regression or normalisation of tissue; they may be seen in dermatophyte infection or discoid lupus erythematosus.

- **discoid:** a filled circle, e.g. psoriasis
- **arcuate:** incomplete circles (**Figure 2.7**)

Colour	Examples
Black	Melanin, e.g. some naevi, melanoma
	Exogenous pigments, e.g. tattoos, pencil/ink
	Exogenous chemicals, e.g. silver nitrate, gold salts
	Deeply situated blood or melanin, e.g. angiomas, blue naevus
Blue–grey	Inflammatory diseases, e.g. orf
	Drug-induced pigmentation, e.g. phenothiazines, minocycline
Dark brown	Melanin nearest the skin surface, mostly melanocytic naevi
	Exogenous pigments, e.g. dithranol (anthralin) staining
Pale brown	Melanin near the skin surface, e.g. lentigo, freckles
Muddy brown	Melanin in the superficial surface, e.g. post-inflammatory pigmentation
Purple	Vascular lesions, e.g. angiomas
Dusky blue	Reduced amounts of oxygenated haemoglobin, e.g. poor arterial supply, central causes of cyanosis, methaemoglobinaemia
Violaceous and lilac	Lichen planus, edge of plaques of morphoea, connective tissue disorders, e.g. dermatomyositis
Pink–red	Many exanthemas and common disorders, e.g. psoriasis
Red–brown	Inflammatory dermatoses, e.g. seborrhoeic eczema, secondary syphilis
	Haemosiderosis, e.g. pigmented purpuric dermatoses

Table 2.4 Causes of skin colour change

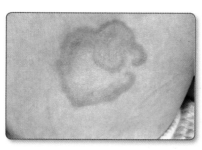

Figure 2.7 Arcuate lesion on a child.

- **serpiginous**: snake-like (**Figure 2.8**)
- **polycyclic**: multiple circles that merge together
- **livedoid**: wide lace-like pattern
- **reticulate**: fine lace-like pattern
- **targetoid**: like an archer's board (**Figure 2.9** and **2.10**)

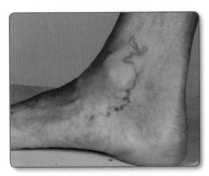

Figure 2.8 Serpiginous lesion of cutaneous larva migrans.

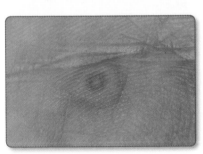

Figure 2.9 Targetoid lesion of erythema multiforme.

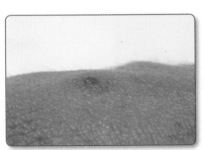

Figure 2.10 Elevation of targetoid lesion on the skin, making the lesion palpable.

Palpate

Palpation of the skin gives further information about the texture, tenderness, temperature and thickness of the skin – the '4Ts':

- Using your index fingers, run your fingers over the lesions and note the surface texture and whether the lesions are elevated or flat. An altered surface texture will be palpated due to the scale in this dermatophyte infection (**Figure 2.11**).
- Gently, without causing pain, press on the lesion to determine the consistency – firm, fluctuant or soft.
- Note how deep the lesion is – whether it is tethered and fixed to the dermis or deeper and freely mobile.
- The temperature of the eruption should be noted.
- A gentle scratch of the skin may reveal 'dermographism' (**Figure 2.12**).
- A gentle push into the skin with the index and middle finger can assess for oedema.

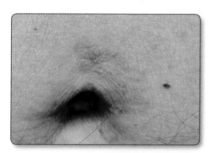

Figure 2.11 Altered surface texture due to scale in a periumbilical dermatophyte infection.

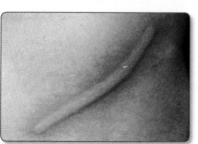

Figure 2.12 Dermographism.

2.4 Dermatological investigations

To confirm the diagnosis from a list of differential diagnoses after the history and examination, further investigation is usually required. Special investigations may also be required to subdefine the diagnosis, such as genotyping, which will give a more precise prognosis and therapeutic options for the disease. The most common special investigations are described below, with details of how they are performed and the dermatoses for which you should be using them.

Microbial identification
Skin swabs

These are used if you suspect or wish to exclude a bacterial or viral infection.
- Dip the swab into the culture medium and then rub it onto the skin for the highest yield.

Mycology

Skin scrapings and nail clippings are taken to exclude or confirm the diagnosis of a fungal infection by microscopy and culture.
- Take a sample from the leading edge of the rash.
- Use one of the following methods: scrape the skin with the dull side of the blade, use adhesive tape gently applied to the skin, use a toothbrush to collect scale from the scalp, or take nail clippings and debris from the distal nail plate.
- Potassium hydroxide is added to dissolve the keratinocytes, which are then stained and viewed under the microscope.
- Culture may take several weeks at 25–30°C.

Wood's lamp

This is an ultraviolet light that has a nickel oxide filter to remove nearly all visible rays; the test is performed to help detect the presence of some infections, variations in epidermal melanin or the deposition/presence of porphyrins (**Figure 2.13** and **Table 2.5**):
- The patient is taken to a dark room. The Wood's lamp is held 10–15 cm from the area being examined. Avoid shining the light directly into the patient's eyes.

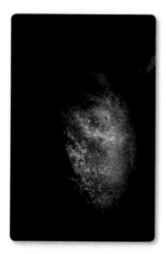

Figure 2.13 Wood's light causes *Corynebacterium* in erythrasma to fluoresce a coral red colour.

Colour under Wood's light	Disease
Coral red	*Corynebacterium minutissimum* (erythrasma) (**Figure 2.13**)
Pale green	*Trichophyton schoenleinii*
Blue	*Pseudomonas aeruginosa*
Pink–orange	Porphyria cutanea tarda
Ash-leaf white spot	Tuberous sclerosis
Bright white	Vitiligo

Table 2.5 Colour of fluorescence under Wood's light

- Deodorants, make-up and recent washing of the skin may give a false-negative result.

Skin imaging
Dermatoscopy
Dermatoscopy is a non-invasive method that allows the in vivo evaluation of colours and microstructures of the epidermis and the papillary dermis. It is mainly used to evaluate pigmented skin lesions. The dermatoscope (**Figure 2.14**) is a simple,

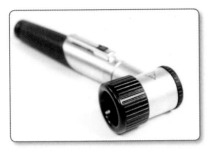

Figure 2.14 The dermatoscope is used to aid lesion identification.

user-friendly tool that utilises illuminations and ×10 magnification. It is used primarily to improve melanoma detection, but is also useful in the detection of other skin tumours and scabies infection. The method of use is as follows.

- The lesion is covered in a drop of oil; this enhances the transparency of the stratum corneum.
- The dermatoscope is placed on the skin and the colours and the pattern are noted; analysis of these factors points towards a diagnosis.

Reflectance confocal microscopy

Reflectance confocal microscopy (RCM) allows for in vivo skin imaging at cellular resolution to the depth of the papillary dermis and in real time. It uses a near-infrared laser light, which is focused on a microscopic skin target and reflected to re-form the magnified image. RCM is primarily used for skin cancer detection, but is increasingly used as an alternative to traditional histopathology (**Figure 2.15**).

Light microscopy

Simple microscopy is useful for the detection of hair shaft abnormalities and fungal detection.

Allergic investigations
Skin-prick tests

These tests are used to determine the cause of internal allergy, not contact allergy.

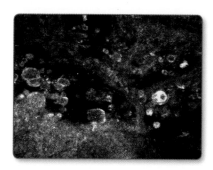

Figure 2.15 Reflectance confocal imaging of the skin: large, bright, white, round structures are melanoma cells.

- Suspected causes of allergy are mixed with liquid to make a solution, which is then dropped on to the skin.
- The skin beneath is then pricked with a needle.
- A positive reaction is seen if the skin becomes erythematous or forms a weal in 20 min.

Radioallergosorbent test

This is particularly useful for young children or patients in whom there may be a risk with prick testing. It is a measure of circulating antibodies to allergens and correlates well with skin-prick testing.

> **Clinical insight**
>
> Antihistamines and corticosteroids should not be taken before allergy testing due to the likelihood of creating a false-negative result.

Patch tests (Figure 2.16)

These are used in patients with dermatitis to determine which chemical may be causing or exacerbating it. A range of substances can be used. A positive test is noted if the area beneath a chemical has a reaction ranging from a pale, raised, pink weal to blistering and ulceration. The method is as follows.

- At the initial appointment, chemicals are applied to the back with special adhesive tape.
- Two days later the patches are removed and the back is examined.
- A further 2 days later the back is examined and any reaction noted.

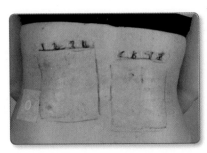

Figure 2.16 Patch testing: the patient has tested positive to the chemical at the top of column 1.

Phototests

Phototests are used to confirm the presence of an abnormal sunburn reaction. The investigation is done in highly specialised units and performed using a monochromator.

Blood tests

Blood tests are used in dermatology less frequently than in other areas of medicine. They are used when systemic disease is expected, to monitor systemic disease progress or levels of a drug, e.g. ciclosporin. Blood may also be taken for genotyping to further define a disease.

Blood tests are often used as part of a screen to try to determine a systemic cause for a dermatological symptom or sign.

Pruritus screen

A typical screen for pruritus should include:

- full blood count (FBC) and serum ferritin – iron-deficiency anaemia, polycythaemia and leukaemia may all cause pruritus
- eosinophils – these may be raised in allergy and a number of other conditions (**Table 2.6**)
- fasting blood glucose
- liver function tests (LFTs) – if raised, functional enzymes may cause itch
- renal function and electrolytes – for cases of itch in renal failure
- thyroid function tests – hypothyroidism or hyperthyroidism may cause systemic pruritus

Eosinophilia in dermatology patients
Atopic disorders: eczema, asthma, hay fever
Parasitic infections: scabies, worms
Malignancy: Hodgkin's disease, leukaemia
Bullous disease: pemphigus, dermatitis herpetiformis
Hypereosinophilic syndrome

Table 2.6 Causes of eosinophilia in dermatology patients

Vasculitis screen

A patient presenting with signs of vasculitis should have a dip test urinalysis for blood and protein and a chest radiograph; he or she should also undergo the following tests:

- FBC
- renal function and electrolytes
- LFTs
- inflammatory markers
- hepatitis serology [types B and C are associated with panarteritis nodosa and mixed cryoglobulinaemia, respectively]
- cryoglobulins
- complement levels
- HIV test
- rheumatoid factor
- antinuclear antibodies (ANAs)

Autoantibody screen

A patient may present with systemic symptoms including myalgia, arthralgia and a widespread rash, and an autoantibody screen may be performed.

- ANAs:
  - these include double-stranded DNA (dsDNA), anti-histone, anti-centromere and Mi-2
  - ANAs at a titre of 1:40 are present in 32% of the general population
  - chronic illness and smoking can lead to ANA positivity

- extractable nuclear antigens (ENAs):
  - antigens within the nucleus
  - main antigens are Ro, La, RNP, Sm, Jo-1 and Scl-70

The importance of ANA/ENA profiles can be seen when a typical pattern points towards or confirms a diagnosis, particularly in systemic lupus erythematosus (SLE). Up to 100% of patients with SLE will be positive for ANAs and the presence of dsDNA. Anti-Sm, anti-Jo-1, anti-RNP, anti-Ro and anti-La may also be present. In 95% of patients with drug-induced lupus there may be positivity for anti-histone antibodies. Anti-Scl-70 is the most frequent finding in diffuse morphoea, and anti-centromere in localised morphoea. Autoantibody testing is particularly useful in dermatomyositis because different antibody profiles indicate different disease associations and hence different management plans, e.g. anti-TIF-1γ is associated with severe cutaneous changes, myositis and an increased risk of internal malignancy.

Cold-induced conditions

Patients with significant cold-induced disorders and associated tissue damage should, in addition to a vasculitis screen, have an investigation for cryoproteins.

For this the blood sample is taken and placed in a vacuum flask to keep it at a temperature of 37°C until it reaches the laboratory.

Tissue examination

Dermatopathology

Skin biopsy and histopathology are generally thought to be the gold standard for diagnosis. Skin biopsy specimens are processed by fixing them in paraffin, then staining with haematoxylin and eosin (H&E). With this stain, eosinophilic or acidic structures stain red, whereas basophilic or alkaline structures stain blue. Occasionally, special stains may be requested to see bacteria, fungi or substances deposited in the skin, such as amyloid or iron. Additional tests may be performed on biopsy specimens, using immunohistochemistry. This technique allows detection of antigens in tissue sections, using labelled antibodies. The marker may be a fluorescent dye, enzyme system or radioactive element. It is used predominantly for malignant tumours.

The specimen is systematically examined by looking at the structure of the epidermis, dermis, subcutis and fascia to the depth of the tissue. From the results of this examination, a list of differential and definitive diagnoses can be made and a report issued.

Dermatopathology, as with other aspects of dermatology, has its own terminology, which is commonly used in reports. Some of the more common findings are noted here to help interpretation and provide the terminology for common findings seen on H&E staining.

Inflammatory conditions

The following changes are seen:

- epidermal changes:
  - **hyperkeratosis**: thickening of the stratum corneum
  - **parakeratosis**: nuclei within the stratum corneum
  - **acanthosis**: thickened squamous cell layer
  - **spongiosis**: intercellular oedema between keratinocytes
  - **exocytosis**: inflammatory cells within the epidermis
  - **acantholysis**: keratinocyte separation due to loss of cell adhesion
  - **lichenoid**: lymphocytes attack the basal epidermis; a band-like pattern is seen
- dermal changes:
  - **dermal atrophy**: thinning of the dermis
  - **oedema**: interstitial fluid in the dermis
  - **hyalinisation**: dense red/pink acellular material
  - **solar elastosis**: bluish stranding in the upper dermis of photo-aged skin
  - **perivascular**: inflammatory cells clustered around blood vessels
  - **haemosiderin**: brown pigment from degraded red blood cells

Inflammatory dermatoses cause histopathological changes that form recognisable tissue reaction patterns. These are based on the epidermal changes and basic pattern of inflammatory cell infiltration. The common patterns are discussed below.

Eczema (Figure 2.17) Eczema can present as:

- spongiosis with associated lymphocyte exocytosis in acute eczema
- acanthosis in chronic eczema
- parakeratosis and occasionally a perivascular lymphohistiocytic infiltrate

Psoriasis There are different subtypes of psoriasis, but the typical changes of chronic plaque psoriasis are:

- hyperkeratosis
- parakeratosis
- Munro's microabscesses – neutrophils in stratum corneum
- regular acanthosis
- dilated capillaries in dermal papillae

Skin tumours When examining cutaneous tumours under light microscopy with H&E staining, the following descriptive words are commonly used:

- dysplastic cells: nuclear enlargement, pleomorphism, nuclear hyperchromatism and atypical mitoses
- basaloid cells: cells from the basal epidermal layer
- epithelioid cells: cells resembling keratinocytes
- spindle cells: different cell types but appearing long and thin
- horn cysts: whorling keratinocytes, more keratinised in the middle
- epidermotropism: malignant cells moving into the epidermis
- pagetoid spread: individual cell spread along the epidermis

Actinic keratosis This can involve:

- hyperkeratosis

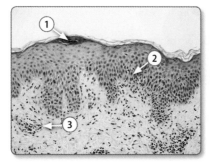

Figure 2.17 Typical histology of eczema. ① Parakeratosis. ② Spongiosis in acute eczema, with associated lymphocyte exocytosis. ③ Perivascular lymphohistiocytic infiltrate.

- columns of parakeratosis
- dysplastic keratinocytes scattered throughout
- superficial perivascular inflammatory infiltrate

Basal cell carcinoma (BCC) shows **(Figure 2.18):**
- cohesive nests of basaloid tumour cells
- peripheral palisading of nuclei at the margins
- retraction noted around the edges of the nests
- stromal reaction

Direct immunofluorescence

Some dermatoses, such as pemphigus, pemphigoid and dermatitis herpetiformis, also benefit from an additional sample being taken and sent for direct immunofluorescence. A punch biopsy of the skin is taken and placed on gauze soaked in saline, put in a dry pot and sent for same-day processing. The technique uses a single antibody, directed to the known antigen, which is chemically linked to a fluorophore. The fluorophore that it carries can be detected with the fluorescence microscope **(Figure 2.19)**.

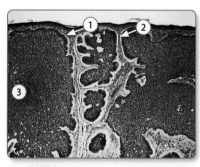

Figure 2.18 Typical histology of basal cell carcinoma. ① Peripheral palisading. ② Retraction. ③ Nest of tumour cells.

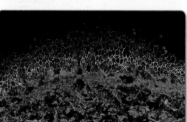

Figure 2.19 Direct IgG immunofluorescence in pemphigus vulgaris.

Dermatology nursing and therapeutics

The demands on and the skills and knowledge base required by the dermatology nurse have changed dramatically in recent years, because hospital admission levels are lower with the availability of more effective creams, phototherapy and oral immunosuppressive agents, and most treatments are now carried out on an outpatient basis. Within these outpatient settings the dermatology nurse has a key role in patient education, wound care and the application of topical therapies.

Before starting any topical treatments it is important to:
- make a diagnosis
- take a holistic approach
- ensure that the patient understands the diagnosis, treatment plan and side effects
- ensure that the patient will be able to comply with treatment
- explain the difference between control and cure for chronic disease

3.1 Topical therapies

Topical agents are the most common treatments used in dermatology; correct application is required to ensure the medication's efficacy. This must be explained clearly to the patient, usually after the prescribing physician or nurse has demonstrated an initial application.

Topical treatments vary depending on the dermatosis, and its site and severity. The treatments contain two components:
1. The active drug
2. The carrier medium (base)

Both are required for optimal efficacy; the carrier medium affects the degree of hydration of the skin, has a mild anti-inflammatory effect and helps penetration of the active drug.

It is important to know which base is appropriate for which sites and conditions. **Table 3.1** highlights the differences and indications for use.

Carrier medium	Content	Use and effectiveness	Pros and cons
Gels 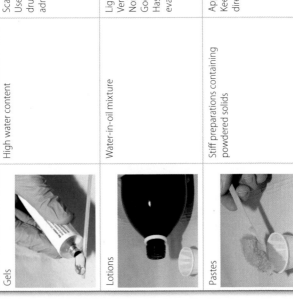	High water content	Scalp and hairy areas Useful for suspending insoluble drugs and facilitating their administration and absorption	Quickly evaporates effect. Limited moisturising
Lotions	Water-in-oil mixture	Light weight Very easy to apply over large areas Non-greasy Good for areas of broken skin Has a cooling effect from evaporation	Limited long-term moisturising effect Will need frequent applications
Pastes	Stiff preparations containing powdered solids	Apply directly to a specific lesion Keeps the active ingredient directly on the area of application	Needs to be removed with liquid paraffin

Carrier medium	Content	Use of effectiveness	Pros and cons
Creams	Emulsions of water and oil	Easy to apply Cooling Good for broken and weepy skin	Medium moisturising; not appropriate for very dry skin Can contain preservatives which are potential sensitisers
Ointments	Oil based	Very greasy and occlusive Very moisturising Excellent for dry skin Adds moisture as well as trapping moisture in Do not contain preservatives	Also traps heat, which can cause itching if the skin gets too hot Greasiness can feel uncomfortable for the patient Grease stains clothes Patients needs to avoid getting into eyes

Table 3.1 Carrier media of topical agents

3.2 Topical agents

These agents include:

- moisturisers (emollients)
- corticosteroids
- vitamin D derivatives
- calcineurin inhibitors
- cytotoxic agents

Moisturisers (emollients)

The terms 'moisturiser' (to add moisture) and 'emollient' (to soften) are often interchangeable, so they can be confusing, but their main actions are:

- **occlusive**: a layer of oil on the surface of the skin slows water loss
- **humectant**: they bind and hold water in the stratum corneum at high concentrations

Thorough assessment of the skin will indicate which type of moisturiser should be applied, and where. The aim is to have soft, flexible, non-scaly skin which is comfortable for the patient. This prevents water loss and skin cracking, thereby reducing inflammation, itching and the subsequent risk of infection.

Patients with very dry skin will need oily preparations; patients with less severe dryness will need a water-based preparation more.

In chronic conditions, continuous use of a moisturising regimen is advised even if the condition appears to be fully treated; this is to:

- maintain the protective barrier of the skin and reduce recurrence
- prepare the skin to receive other topical treatments, such as topical steroids

Table 3.2 shows how to apply moisturisers. Reapplication is recommended before the skin gets dry. If the condition is severe, e.g. erythrodermic psoriasis, 2-hourly applications are necessary. In contrast, once a day may be adequate in patients with eczema that is cared for well.

Moisturising maintenance regimen with correct application	
· Wash with soap substitute; avoid perfumed soaps because they may irritate	
· Baths: add oil to water, which deposits a layer of oil on the skin when rising out of the bath	
· Showers: avoid long hot showers or baths because they dry the skin	

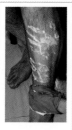	Pat the skin gently but not completely; do not rub – this can irritate the skin Apply moisturiser with your hands; pat equal amounts over the affected area	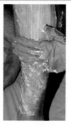	Smooth in downward strokes, in the direction of hair follicles
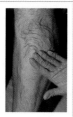	Do not rub in; this can force cream into the follicles and cause folliculitis	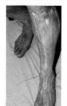	The moisturiser should be evident on the skin (the skin should glisten). Allow the moisturiser to be completely absorbed (about 30 min) before applying topical steroids; this avoids diluting the steroid and ensures good skin preparation to absorb the treatment

Table 3.2 Application of an emollient

Topical corticosteroids

Steroids are anti-inflammatories; they have immunosuppressive qualities, are vasoconstrictive and have an antimitotic effect.

They have revolutionised disease treatment in dermatology.

- They are available in different strengths (**Table 3.3**) .
- Antifungals and antimicrobials can be added for use in combination with the steroid.

Topical steroids are used to treat inflammatory exacerbations, and the following rules should be followed.

- Use the most effective strength of steroid to control the disease quickly and safely. This should then be stepped down to a less potent steroid once the disease is under control
- Patients should be reviewed after 1 week following a flare, and regularly if using potent steroids
- Reassure parents and carers about the benefits of topical steroids when used appropriately, as well as explaining the side effects when used inappropriately
- Use a growth chart for children

Potent steroids should be used in infants with extreme caution, particularly in the nappy area, due to the risk of systemic absorption.

Application

Topical steroids can be applied once a day, at night-time. Patients should be advised to apply the moisturiser first and allow it to be completely absorbed before applying the steroid. The amount sufficient to cover the adult body once is 15 g. To help achieve the correct dosage, the number of 'finger-tip units' (FTUs) are recorded. An FTU is the amount of cream squeezed

Therapeutic strength	Steroid	Site
Weak	Hydrocortisone (HC)	Face and flexures
Moderately potent	Clobetasone butyrate (25× strength of HC)	Body
Potent	Betamethasone valerate (100× strength of HC)	Body
Very potent	Clobetasol propionate (600× strength of HC)	Not on the face or flexures

Table 3.3 Topical steroid gradient of strength

from a tube on to the index finger, from tip to distal interphalangeal joint (**Figure 3.1**). It is a very useful unit to discuss when
educating patients; the average FTU provides 0.5 g cream or
coverage the size of one hand, allowing patients to calculate
the correct dose for the body area (**Figure 3.2**).

Side effects of topical steroids

The risk of side effects depends on the strength of the steroid,
length of application, site treated and nature of the skin prob-

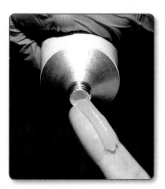

Figure 3.1 The fingertip unit (FTU).

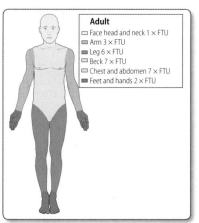

Adult
- Face head and neck 1 × FTU
- Arm 3 × FTU
- Leg 6 × FTU
- Beck 7 × FTU
- Chest and abdomen 7 × FTU
- Feet and hands 2 × FTU

Figure 3.2 Fingertip unit
(FTU): quantity per body
area (adult).

lem. Areas of thin skin, such as the face, skinfolds and genitalia, and areas with a high density of follicles, such as the axilla and scalp, absorb the steroid rapidly. Absorption is increased in areas under occlusive dressings such as hydrocolloid and polythene. The addition of urea or salicylic acid to the steroid also enhances absorption. This increased absorption will cause an increase in local side effects, such as flushing and skin thinning (**Figure 3.3**).

Steroid resistance may develop and there may be side effects, especially if occlusive therapy has been used. Side effects include:

- skin atrophy
- telangiectasia
- striae
- easy bruising
- acne
- perioral dermatitis

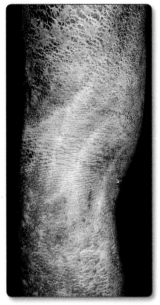

Figure 3.3 Atrophy of the skin on the arm due to excess steroid use. Note the background chronic underlying eczema with lichenification.

Cushing's syndrome has been reported as a result of extensive cutaneous absorption.

Calcineurin inhibitors

Calcineurin inhibitors (0.03% and 0.1% tacrolimus and 1% pimecrolimus) are topical immunomodulators that reduce inflammation via T-cell suppression. They are the second-line treatment for moderate-to-severe eczema not controlled by topical corticosteroids. The side effects include skin irritation, erythema, infections and photosensitivity.

Vitamin D derivatives

As the first-line topical treatment for psoriasis, vitamin D analogues suppress keratinocyte proliferation and induce epidermal differentiation. They should not be used in erythrodermic or pustular psoriasis. Benefits are seen 8–12 weeks after initiation of treatment. Hypercalcaemia may occur if the dose exceeds 100 g/week.

Antitumoral agents

Topical 5-fluorouracil

5-Fluorouracil is a cytotoxic antimetabolite used in the treatment of premalignant skin lesions and low-risk basal cell carcinomas. Dysplastic and malignant cells in the treated area die. It is important to ensure that patients are fully aware of the inflammatory response that will appear 1 week after starting treatment, continuing until 1 week after completion of treatment. Patient information should be given to explain that the inflammatory response is caused by dysplastic cell death and a contact dermatitis or skin infection.

Imiquimod 5%

This is a topical immunomodulator that is effective against neoplastic or premalignant lesions. The local immunity and inflammation are increased, with destruction of the damaged cells. It is imperative that patient information and a contact number be given, because of the brisk inflammatory response that the patient may develop. A small percentage of patients will complain of flu-like symptoms and tiredness, which resolve on stopping the medication.

Patient safety with topical agents

The following must be done to ensure patient safety.

- Decant moisturisers into a separate pot before use, because it is possible to cause microbial contamination of the product.
- Occlusive moisturisers can trap heat in the skin, causing irritation and increased itch.
- Folliculitis can be a side effect of occlusive moisturisers and incorrect application of topical agents. If applied in the opposite direction to the hair follicles they can cause or exacerbate facial acne.
- Patients should be advised not to smoke tobacco products if they have bandages with ointment bases.
- Patient information leaflets should be given to the patient, together with any treatment plan.

3.3 Occlusive dressings

Occlusive dressings, such as wet wrapping or paste bandaging, can intensify the treatment and enhance efficiency by restricting transepidural water loss and increasing hydration. Prevention of direct access to the skin can prevent the patient from scratching and introducing infection. Occlusive dressings can intensify the efficacy and absorption of topical steroids, which can also increase the risk of steroid-induced side effects.

Medicated paste bandaging is excellent for weepy infected areas; it can hold medication close to the skin for maximum effect. A folded or pleated technique should be used to allow the bandage to contract, avoiding constriction of the limb when evaporation occurs (**Figure 3.4**).

An occlusive plastic wrap on the scalp can help to lift off encrusted psoriasis plaques or ensure that treatments in awkward places such as the feet are kept in place.

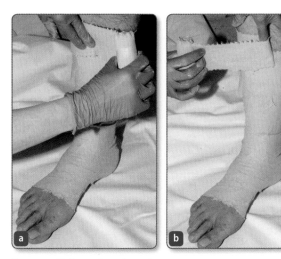

Figure 3.4 Technique for occlusive dressing.

3.4 Topical agents for wound care

Acute and chronic wounds are a major cause of morbidity. Early correct management of these can greatly improve a patient's quality of life. Acute wounds may be caused by trauma or be iatrogenic. Appropriate care can reduce the rate of complications and speed up wound healing. Chronic skin wounds are commonly ulcers resulting from pressure, venous stasis or diabetes mellitus.

Acute wounds

Basic wound healing goes through several stages (**Figure 3.5**):

- haemostatic
- inflammatory
- proliferative
- contraction
- re-epithelialisation
- remodelling

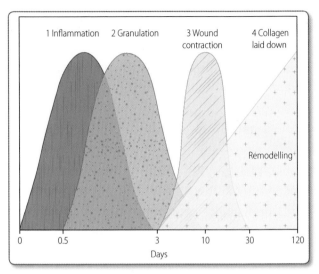

Figure 3.5 The key stages of basic wound healing.

Haemostatic

This stage involves the following.

- Blood clotting acts as a matrix for cell migration.
- Release of growth factors is needed for wound healing.

Inflammatory

Wound cleaning and release of growth factors occur.

- Inflammation results from increased blood flow and fluid in tissues.
- Neutrophils mop up bacteria and debris.
- Exudate bathes the wound site and acts as a transport medium for healing cells.

Proliferative

Growth of new cells and formation of granulation tissue occur. Macrophages and lymphocytes clean the wound bed and produce transforming growth factor, which promotes formation of new tissue and blood vessels, and fibroblast growth factor, which stimulates growth of fibroblasts that in turn stimulate healing.

Contraction

After formation of granulation tissue, fibroblasts congregate on wound margins and contraction of the wound starts.

Re-epithelialisation

Epithelial cells grow from the margins.

Remodelling

Collagen fibres increase in strength.
- Redness is lost, as an increased blood supply is no longer required.
- Scar tissue changes over time may occur for up to 2 years.

Dressings

Optimal wound healing occurs in a moist environment with occlusion; this can be achieved by using petrolatum ointment and one of the many occlusive or semiocclusive dressings, e.g. hydrocolloid, alginates, hydrogels and foam dressings. The main aims of dressings are to:
- produce rapid and cosmetically acceptable healing
- prevent infection
- debride dead tissue/slough and contain exudate
- reduce pain

Post-surgical wound care

Biopsies and minor surgery are common occurrences in dermatology, especially on the face when dealing with skin cancer.

Large sutured wounds These need a pressure dressing for 24–48 hours, depending on bleeding risk. They are then kept clean, moist and covered, until the sutures have been removed. It is necessary to:
- **clean** with normal soap and water
- **keep moist** with ointment applied to sutures using a clean finger

- **keep covered** with waterproof dressing to avoid scab formation and prevent infection

  Dressings should be changed every 24 hours to assess the wound for infection.

Granulating wounds These will take longer to heal and must be kept clean, moist and covered until they are completely healed; this may take weeks, depending on the size and site of the wound. Scab formation should be avoided because this can impede wound healing, obscure assessment and hide infection.

Lower leg wounds Such wounds, especially on elderly people or those with circulatory deficiency, may benefit from application of a tubular pressure dressing.

3.5 Chronic wounds

Venous hypertension in the lower legs can cause changes in the microcirculation of the skin of the distal extremity; this can lead to chronic dermatitis and non-healing ulceration.

Stasis dermatitis

Stasis dermatitis is a common inflammatory skin disease that occurs on the lower extremities. It is usually the earliest cutaneous sequela of chronic venous insufficiency with venous hypertension, and a precursor to venous leg ulceration. Patients will have pruritus and discoloration (usually brown/red from haemosiderin deposition), and the skin may have a cobblestone texture. The patient may also present with red, acutely painful lower legs (**Figure 3.6**). The fact that this condition is bilateral is a key difference from lower leg cellulitis, which is usually unilateral.

Management

Management involves:

- using class 1 or 2 compression stockings
- avoiding standing still for long periods of time
- elevating the legs when sitting or lying down
- using an emollient

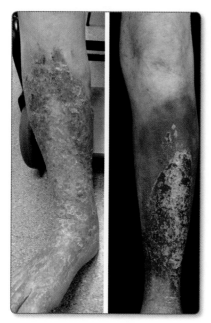

Figure 3.6 Acute and chronic stasis dermatitis in the same patient.

- using steroid ointment – mild/moderate, depending on severity and occlusion

Venous leg ulceration

With continued compromise to the microcirculation, skin ulceration can occur, typically on the medial distal leg but it may be circumferential (**Figure 3.7**).

Management

To manage venous leg ulceration:
- ensure there is a competent arterial supply incompetence (ankle–brachial pressure index >0.8)
- exclude other causes of leg ulcers, for example:
  - diabetic ulcers
  - infection

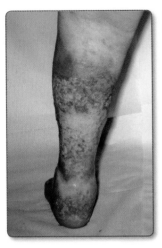

Figure 3.7 Superficial venous ulceration and contact dermatitis.

- – vasculitis
- – skin cancer

Graduated compression and elevation of the extremity are the mainstay of treatment.

Compression

Graduated compression is achieved using a four-layer technique or compression stockings. Class 3 compression bandages are the ones most commonly used to treat active ulcers.

Compression bandages As a four-layer technique these can sustain high pressure for a considerable time and allow for a weekly change of dressings:

- layer 1: orthopaedic wool
- layer 2: crepe bandage
- layer 3: elastic bandage
- layer 4: elastic cohesive bandage

The patient should understand that this can initially be painful. Analgesia and an adjustment in lifestyle may be required to facilitate healing.

Further interventions include ablation of incompetent truncal veins with laser or radiofrequency, and use of sclerosant injections to close incompetent perforator veins.

3.6 Systemic agents in dermatology

Antibiotics

Oral doses and occasionally intravenous doses of antibiotics are required to treat infections and inflammatory conditions such as acne.

- Streptococcal infections: flucloxacillin is the drug of choice (erythromycin if the patient is penicillin allergic).
- Streptococcal infections: benzylpenicillin is the drug of choice.
- Inflammatory disease (acne/rosacea): low-dose tetracyclines are first-line treatment.

Antifungal agents

Systemic treatment is usually required for resistant skin disease and for most hair and nail infections:

- **Terbinafine** is a highly effective fungicide for most dermatophytes.
- **Griseofulvin** is less expensive than terbinafine and useful for the scalp.

Antihistamines

Antihistamines block the histamine receptors. In dermatology H_1-receptor antihistamines are most effective. They may be:

- **non-sedating**: loratadine/cetirizine – often used in patients with allergy or urticaria
- **sedating**: chlorphenamine/hydroxyzine – often used at night-time to enable a patient to sleep

Retinoids

Retinoids are derivatives of vitamin A: they are used to treat acne (isotretinoin) and psoriasis (acitretin) and to prevent skin cancer in transplant recipients (acitretin). They are teratogenic. Women should not become pregnant while taking isotretinoin, and acitretin should not be used within 2 years of a planned pregnancy. Side effects of treatment include:

- dryness of the mucosal membranes, particularly the lips
- musculoskeletal aches and pains
- rise in serum triglycerides

- poor wound healing
- reversible hair loss

Systemic steroids

Systemic steroids should be used only under supervision by a dermatologist, because many diseases flare on the introduction or cessation of systemic steroid therapy. For many of the blistering and autoantibody-mediated diseases, they are essential. The side effects of systemic steroids are well described (**Table 3.4**). Patients have very regular check-ups to prevent complications.

Immunosuppressive agents

These drugs should be used only under the supervision of a dermatologist.

- **Methotrexate**: inhibits cell division; used in the treatment of psoriasis. It is teratogenic. Regular blood tests are required to monitor for bone marrow suppression and liver fibrosis. Patients should take a folic acid supplement.

Acute (<1 month)
Sleep disturbance
Increase in appetite
Psychosis
Weight gain
Long term
Skin: acne, atrophy, hypertrichosis, alopecia
Redistribution of body fat: buffalo hump, moon face, central obesity
Eye: glaucoma, cataracts
Gastrointestinal tract: ulceration, hepatic steatosis
Cardiovascular: increased risk of myocardial infarction, stroke
Metabolic: increased risk of diabetes
Nervous system: headaches, tremor

Table 3.4 Side effects of systemic steroids

- **Ciclosporin**: immunosuppressive agent used in eczema and psoriasis. It is not teratogenic. Regular tests are required to monitor for nephrotoxicity and hypertension.
- **Azathioprine**: used for eczema and psoriasis and blistering disorders. It is teratogenic. Monitoring is required for myelosuppression.
- **Biologic therapies**: given via subcutaneous injection or intravenous infusion. Theses agents target specific parts of the immune system disease pathway rather than the immune system as a whole. In psoriasis, commonly blocking proteins in the immune system are tumour necrosis factor-α (TNF-α) and interleukins 12 and 23. Monitoring is required for immunosuppression.

Phototherapy

Many dermatoses improve in response to exposure to ultraviolet (UV) radiation; this is reproduced by artificial lights in booths, using light from the appropriate area of the spectrum (**Figure 3.8**).

UVA (320–400 nm) is used, together with a psoralen, for the effective treatment of a number of conditions (**Figure 3.8**). The psoralen sensitises the patient to the UVA light and can be administered orally or topically. Side effects include an increase in skin ageing, non-melanoma skin cancers and cataracts.

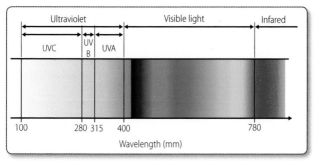

Figure 3.8 Spectrum of light.

UVB (280–315 nm) is used (**Figure 3.8**); more specifically, for psoriasis a narrower band of treatment TL-01 (311–313 nm) is more effective and safer.

3.7 Patient education and health promotion

Every opportunity should be taken to empower patients with knowledge about their condition. This must be tailored to a patient's needs and level of understanding; not all patients can understand the intricacies of their treatment and condition. If you involve patients, they are more likely to be proactive and compliant with treatments.

Patient information leaflets are available from several sources, for example the British Association of Dermatology website.

Self-examination for patients at high risk of skin cancer should be encouraged (**Table 3.5**).

Examine the entire face – use mirrors for behind the ear
Inspect the scalp using a hair dryer and mirror
Check the hands – palms, dorsum, fingernails
Check the arms including the axillae
Check the neck, chest and torso, including under the breasts
Examine the back – using full-length and hand mirrors
Examine the buttocks and backs of the legs
Examine the front of the legs and feet, plantar and toes

Table 3.5 Self-examination: guide for patients at high risk of skin cancer

Diagnostic pathways

This chapter presents a set of diagnostic flowcharts for some common signs in dermatology. Further flowcharts are included within individual chapters where appropriate.

We suggest that you use the flowcharts in tandem with clinical assessment, e.g. if you are asked to review a patient with blisters, use Figure 4.5 and follow the column with the closest matching clinical signs to reach a diagnosis.

These flowcharts do not deal with an exhaustive set of dermatological conditions but contain many of the common skin diseases that you will encounter in clinical practice.

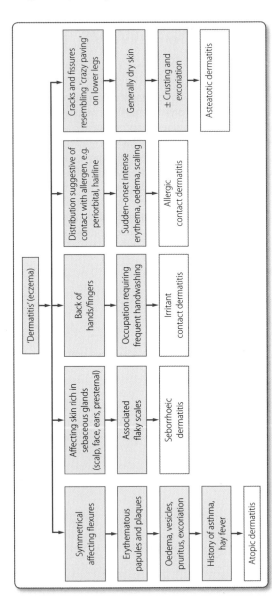

Figure 4.1 Dermatitis.

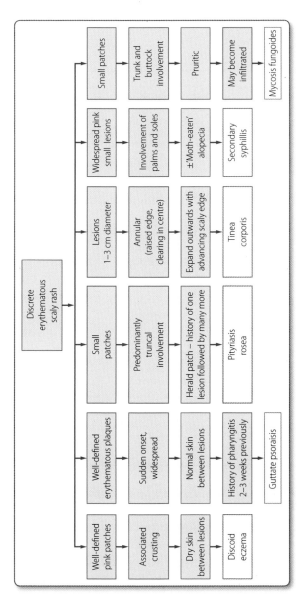

Figure 4.2 Discrete erythematous scaly rash.

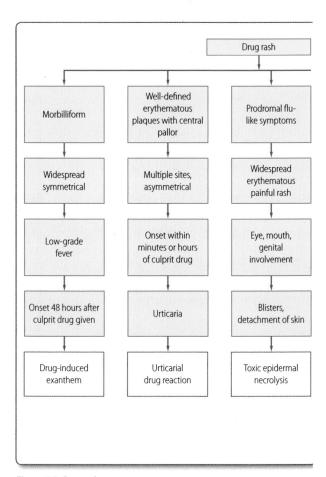

Figure 4.3 Drug rash.
DRESS, drug reaction with eosinophilia and systemic symptoms; LFT, liver function tests.

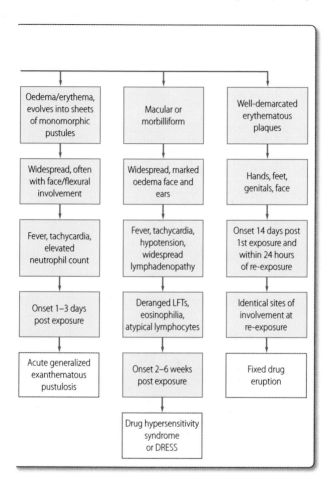

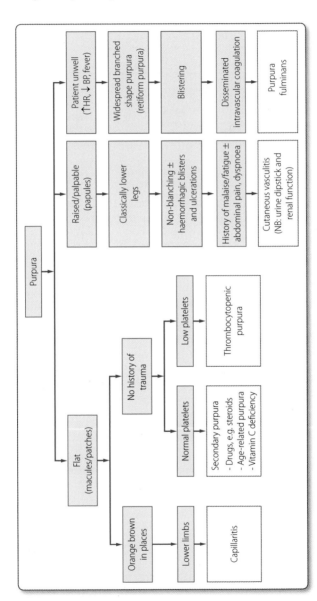

Figure 4.4 Purpura.
BP, blood pressure; HR, heart rate.

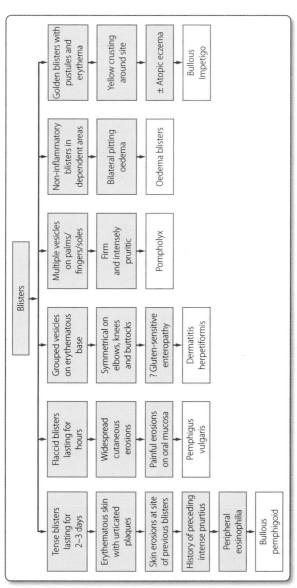

Figure 4.5 Blisters.

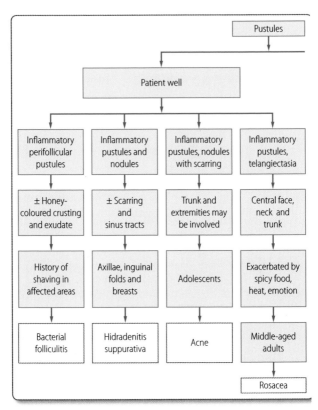

Figure 4.6 Pustules.
HR, heart rate.

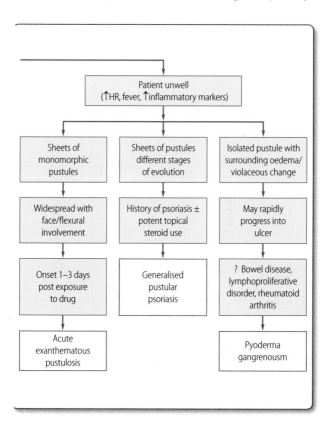

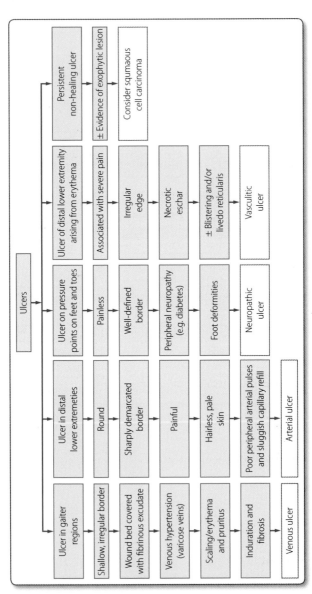

Figure 4.7 Ulcers.

Skin tumours

A skin tumour is an abnormal mass of tissue resulting from aberrant cellular proliferation. The tumour may be benign or malignant. Malignant tumours may be either primary or secondary. Benign disease is more common and represents the bulk of referral of disease and usually requires reassurance and explanation. Skin cancer represents a large burden of disease; its high prevalence and frequent occurrence make it an extremely significant public health problem.

Key points

When assessing a skin tumour it is crucial to bear in mind the following.

- Careful examination, with appropriate use of light and magnification, is required.
- There are specific criteria for the examination of pigmented lesions (**Table 5.1**).
- It is important to identify patients at high risk of skin cancer (**Table 5.2**).

Major features of pigmented lesions (score 2)
Change in size
Irregular shape
Irregular colour
Minor features of pigmented lesions (score 1)
Largest diameter ≥7 mm
Inflammation
Oozing
Change in sensation
Pigmented lesions scoring ≥3 points are suspicious.

Table 5.1 Scoring system for examination of pigmented lesions

High levels of ultraviolet radiation
Outdoor occupation
Outdoor hobbies
Artificial tanning
Cumulative exposure (age)
Burning episodes
Personal risk
Skin phototypes I and II
Family history
Genetic disorders
Previous skin cancer
Immunosuppression
Multiple naevi (>50)

Table 5.2 Features suggesting that an individual is at high risk of developing skin cancer

- Classify lesions as benign only if you have the knowledge to do so; if uncertain, refer or remove the lesion for histo-pathological diagnosis
- In many cases a surgical approach is required for treatment; this is detailed in Chapter 18.

5.1 Clinical scenario

Bleeding nodule on the toe

Presentation

A 32-year-old pregnant woman presents with a 6-week history of a painless, rapidly growing and bleeding nodule on the third toe (**Figure 5.1**). This occurred 3 weeks after a traumatic cut at the same site. She is otherwise well.

Diagnostic approach

A patient presenting with a rapidly growing new lesion on the skin should be assessed for her risk of skin cancer. Make sure

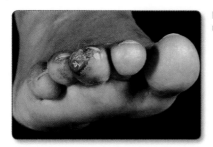

Figure 5.1 Bleeding nodule on the toe.

that you enquire about ultraviolet (UV) exposure, immunosuppression and human papillomavirus (HPV) infections on the fingers. Acral melanomas can occur at this site and are the most common type of melanoma in patients with Fitzpatrick's phototype V and above. The history of previous trauma and pregnancy would suggest a diagnosis of pyogenic granuloma (PG), although in this scenario a melanoma must be excluded.

Examination

The patient has Fitzpatrick's phototype VI. The lesion is a well-demarcated, fleshy, friable nodule with no surrounding pigment network. A full body skin examination reveals no other skin lesions or areas suggestive of photodamage. Lymph node examination is normal.

Diagnostic approach

In any case with a suspicion of malignancy it is important to examine all the skin and regional lymph nodes of the lesion. In this case the characteristics of the lesion are most in keeping with a PG. The main differentials for this lesion are amelanotic melanoma, glomus tumour and squamous cell carcinoma (SCC). Amelanotic melanoma may have a small pigmentary network at the periphery.

Investigations and management

Most PGs are diagnosed by their appearance; however, when in doubt, as in this case, a biopsy of the lesion should be sent for histological examination.

PGs usually occur after minor trauma to the skin as an abnormal wound-healing response. They carry no malignant potential. PGs occurring in pregnancy may resolve; in other cases they tend to persist. They can be removed in several ways (see Chapter 18):

- **complete excision** is the most effective and should be performed if the diagnosis is in doubt
- **curettage and cauterisation**
- **a pulsed dye laser** may be used to shrink small lesions
- **cryotherapy** may be suitable for small lesions

5.2 Benign tumours

Benign tumours are non-cancerous growths on the skin. To differentiate these lesions from more serious entities, it is necessary to appreciate their clinical appearance and the nature of their growth.

Seborrhoeic keratosis

Seborrhoeic keratosis (SK), also termed 'seborrhoeic wart' or 'senile wart' (despite having no viral origin), is very common (**Figure 5.2**). It can occur at any age, but predominantly in middle age, with up to 90% present in patients aged >50 years. Decreases in immunity, but UV radiation and genetics all play a role in their development. Dermatosis papulosa nigra (**Figure 5.3**) is a common variant found on the face of patients with phototypes V and VI.

Clinical features

These common skin tumours may exhibit some or all of the below features.

- SKs may appear on any surface except mucosa and acral surfaces.
- The colour of the lesion varies from light yellow tan to black.
- They may be macular (face and lower legs) or have a rough, 'warty' surface.
- Dermatoscopically, the lesion has a 'stuck-on' appearance, with pearls or cysts embedded in the structure.

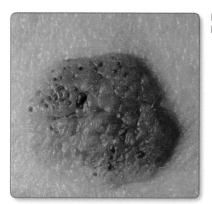

Figure 5.2 Seborrhoeic keratosis.

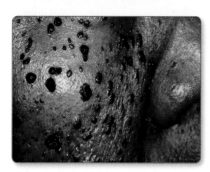

Figure 5.3 Dermatosis papulosa nigra.

- They are usually asymptomatic, but thickened lesions may become itchy.

Treatment

No treatment is necessary unless the lesions become large and troublesome. If removal is indicated then this can be achieved by:

- curettage and cautery
- cryotherapy
- laser surgery

Clinical insight

The Leser–Trélat sign is a sudden onset of multiple seborrhoeic keratoses; it is caused by an associated cancer, usually adenocarcinoma in the gastrointestinal tract.

Freckles

Freckles, also known as ephelides (singular: ephelis), are clusters of concentrated melanin. They can be found in all skin types, but more commonly in light skin, and are related to the presence of the melanocortin-1 receptor gene variant. The formation is triggered by exposure to UVB radiation.

Clinical features

Freckles appear on exposure to sunlight as flat, light brown to red macules; they may fade on reduction of sun exposure.

> **Clinical insight**
>
> Patients with freckling have lower concentrations of protective melanin, and over-exposure to UV radiation should be avoided.

Treatment

No specific treatment is necessary for freckles. Regular use of sunblock can inhibit their development.

Naevi

Naevi (moles) are benign, common growths. They can be hyperpigmented or skin-coloured macules, papules or small plaques. They derive from proliferating melanocytes and develop as a consequence of age, and genetic and environmental factors (e.g. UV exposure).

Naevi are classified by their histological subtype as junctional, compound or intradermal. They may be present at birth (congenital); most develop during childhood and many regress in later life. A tendency to have many ordinary naevi (>50) can be seen in some families.

Clinical features

The characteristics of the different subtypes of naevus are discussed below and depicted in **Figure 5.4**:

- **Junctional naevi** are composed of naevus cells located in the epidermis. They are hyperpigmented macules.
- **Compound naevi** are composed of naevus cells in both the epidermis and the dermis. They are hyperpigmented papules and may be hairy or warty.
- **Intradermal naevi** are similar to compound naevi but usually skin coloured.

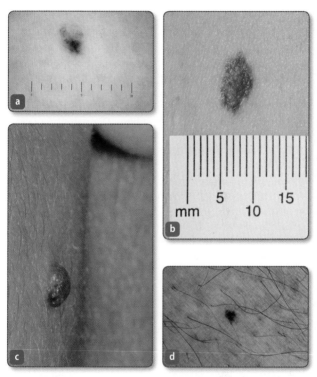

Figure 5.4 Different types of naevi (moles): (a) blue naevus, (b) compound naevus, (c) intradermal naevus and (d) junctional naevus.

- **Blue naevi** have most of their melanocytes in the dermis, and this creates a 'steel blue' colour.

Treatment

No treatment is necessary for these lesions unless they become symptomatic or there is suspicion of malignancy.

For pigmented lesions where there is concern about malignancy, the mole should be fully excised with a 2-mm margin of normal skin.

For removal for cosmetic reasons, lesions may be shave excised, completely excised or removed by laser surgery.

Clinical insight

Halo naevi are moles with a white ring surrounding them. The halo results from an inflammatory process within the naevus. These naevi may be seen more commonly in patients with vitiligo.

Dermatofibroma

A dermatofibroma is a common benign fibrous skin lesion occurring more commonly in women; it frequently develops on the extremities. The aetiology is unknown but may be related to previous insect bites. Dermatofibroma can occur in patients of any age.

Clinical features

Typically dermatofibromas occur as solitary, firm nodules that may be pink to dark brown in colour (**Figure 5.5**); they may be painful.

The 'dimple test' can be performed by squeezing the skin either side of the dermatofibroma; this induces a central dimple to the lesion due to the fibrous lesion tethering down the overlying skin.

Treatment

No treatment is necessary unless there is a concern about the diagnosis or the lesion is painful, in which case the lesion may

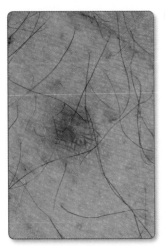

Figure 5.5 Dermatofibroma.

be completely surgically excised. Cryotherapy may be used but this rarely removes the tumour completely.

Lipoma

Lipomas are common, slow-growing tumours of fat cells in the subcutaneous tissue. They occur in 1% of the adult population in both men and women. A blunt injury to the skin may be the trigger for the development of a lipoma.

Clinical features

A lipoma presents as a soft, smooth, rubbery, subcutaneous nodule that moves easily under the skin. The lesion is usually symptomless but some may cause pain (adiposis dolorosa).

Treatment

Most lipomas need no treatment; however, if they are painful they can be removed by one of two methods:
- surgical excision
- punch excision over the central lesion and extrusion of the lipoma

Epidermoid cyst

Epidermoid cysts are common lesions that occur as a consequence of implantation of epidermis into the dermis.

Clinical features

Epidermoid cysts usually:
- are painless, round cysts ranging from 0.5 cm to 5 cm in diameter
- have a central opening that may be plugged and if squeezed will have a thick cheesy discharge (**Figure 5.6**)

Epidermoid cysts may become infected and painful intermittently, and patients often seek medical attention at these times.

Treatment

Cysts that do not cause cosmetic or functional problems

Clinical insight

Epidermoid cysts arise from the epidermis but are often incorrectly referred to as sebaceous cysts. True sebaceous cysts are uncommon and arise from the sebaceous glands.

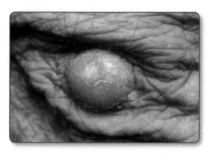

Figure 5.6 Epidermoid cyst.

do not require treatment. If cysts are painful, impair function due to their site or constitute a cosmetic issue, they may be treated with:
- intralesional corticosteroid injections used to reduce inflammation
- complete surgical excision
- punch biopsy and extrusion of cyst contents and the cyst wall

5.3 Categories of skin cancer

The incidence of skin cancers is increasing; it is the most common form of cancer in the UK. Skin cancer can derive from any of the skin structures. They are broadly divided into two categories:
- non-melanoma (derived from basal cells and squamous cells)
- melanoma (derived from melanocytes)

Melanoma and non-melanoma skin cancers account for most skin cancers, with other types making up only a small percentage (**Table 5.3**).

Different skin components react in different ways to UV damage (**Table 5.4**), and this damage may lead to the formation of premalignant lesions. Premalignant lesions of the skin occur commonly in fair skin types in those aged >40 years. These conditions represent in situ disease that may progress to invasive disease.

Skin cancer	Percentage of disease
Basal cell carcinoma	79
Squamous cell carcinoma	17
Malignant melanoma	4
Other: Merkel's cell carcinoma Dermatofibromasarcoma protuberans Adnexal cell tumours Lymphoma	<1

Table 5.3 Categories of skin cancer

Skin component	Consequence of UV damage
Melanocytes	Pigment change, lentigenes
Keratinocytes	Disordered keratin production, actinic keratosis
Collagen	Collagen degradation, altered elastin formation – solar elastosis, wrinkles
Superficial blood vessels	Telangiectasia, bruising

Table 5.4 Consequences of UV damage on skin components

Risk factors

There are multiple risk factors for development of skin cancer including:

Clinical insight

XP is a very rare, autosomal recessive disorder affecting the DNA repair system, resulting in skin cancers, and neurological and eye problems. Freckling or intense sunburn under the age of 2 should prompt consideration of this diagnosis.

- cumulative exposure to UV light
- family history
- episodic sunburn, especially in childhood
- outdoor occupations or hobbies, such as farming and gardening
- Fitzpatrick's skin phototype I and II (see Table 1.1)
- immunosuppression (particularly in renal and cardiac transplant recipients)
- genetic predisposition, e.g. in conditions such as Gorlin's disease and xeroderma pigmentosum (XP)

5.4 Non-melanoma skin cancer

Most non-melanoma skin cancers are related to the level of sun exposure; it is important therefore when examining a patient to record signs of UV damage.

Actinic keratosis

Actinic keratoses (AKs) are areas of epidermal dysplasia, which develop on sun-exposed sites of fair-skinned individuals in response to cumulative sun exposure. In the UK, the prevalence in adults aged >40 years is 11% and for those >70 years, 27%. Long-term immunosuppression (for an organ transplant) is an additional risk factor. The risk of progression to SCC from a single AK is approximately 1%.

Clinical features

Clinical features include:
- erythematous macular lesions, usually with an overlying hyperkeratotic component (**Figure 5.7**)
- usually multiple lesions over an area of UV-induced field change
- occasionally pruritus

Treatment

Treatment for solitary lesions is with either cryotherapy or curettage. If there are multiple lesions in one area, topical treatment with either 5-fluorouracil (5FU) or imiquimod may be given, or the patient may be referred for photodynamic therapy.

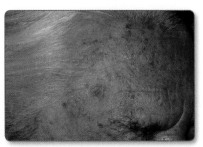

Figure 5.7 Actinic keratosis.

Bowen's disease (SCC in situ)

Bowen's disease represents SCC that is confined within the epidermis with no dermal involvement. Five per cent of

cases are thought to progress to invasive SCC. High-risk sites are the lips and genital areas. The differential diagnoses include eczema, psoriasis, a seborrhoeic wart and a superficial basal cell carcinoma (BCC).

Clinical features

The common clinical features of Bowen's disease are:
- a slowly enlarging, red, scaly patch (**Figure 5.8**)
- occurrence on sun-exposed sites – frequently the lower leg
- lesions that are not typically pruritic

Treatment

If the diagnosis is in doubt, it should be confirmed by biopsy. The treatments are similar to those for actinic keratosis, but in certain instances complete excision may be required.

Basal cell carcinoma

Basal cell carinoma usually occurs in those aged >40 years but are becoming more common in younger patients. BCCs are slow growing and only rarely metastasise. Despite this they can cause considerable damage to local tissues if left untreated. The prognosis, if the condition is diagnosed early and treated correctly, is excellent.

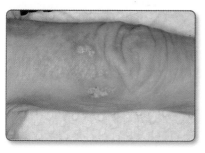

Figure 5.8 Bowen's disease.

Clinical features

BCCs occur at sun-exposed sites, particularly the head and neck (**Figure 5.9**). They present as painless, slow-growing, pale, skin-coloured or red papules that may bleed and never fully heal. The edge of the lesion is pearly; this feature can be made more obvious if the skin overlying the lesion is stretched (**Figure 5.10**).

There are different subtypes with different clinical presentations (**Table 5.5**).

Treatment

A shave biopsy is taken to confirm the diagnosis. After this, a number of treatment options are available and the treatment decision is based on the histology, site and patient choice:

- consider Mohs' micrographic surgery for high-risk BCC (see **Table 5.5**), because it offers the highest cure rate possible – 99%
- surgical excision with a 4-mm margin – 94% cure rate
- radiotherapy – 94% cure rate

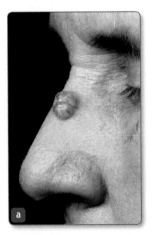
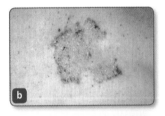
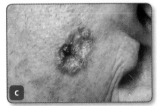

Figure 5.9 (a) Nodular basal cell carcinoma. (b) Superficial basal cell carcinoma. (c) Morphoeic basal cell carcinoma.

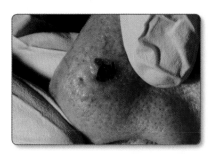

Figure 5.10 Basal cell carcinoma. Note the pearly edge at the distal aspect of the nose that is made more obvious by stretching the skin.

| Tumour size >2 cm |
| Tumour site: nose, perioral, periorbital, ears and hairline |
| Poorly defined edges |
| Histological subtypes: morphoeic, infiltrative, micronodular |
| Recurrent tumour at site of previous treatment |

Table 5.5 Features of high-risk basal cell carcinomas

- cryotherapy
- curettage and cautery
- photodynamic therapy: suitable only for superficial disease
- imiquimod 5% cream and 5FU: suitable only for superficial disease

Clinical insight

Mohs' micrographic surgery (see Figure 18.15) offers the highest possible cure rate for any tumour that is contiguous, e.g. BCC, SCC and dermatofibromasarcoma protuberans (DFSP). This is due to the horizontal processing technique of the tissue, which allows 100% visualisation of the surgical margins.

Squamous cell carcinoma

Squamous cell carcinomas are malignant tumours. They arise from squamous keratinocytes in mucous membranes or the skin epidermis. Unlike BCCs, there is a 5% risk of metastasis. Therefore, a high index of clinical suspicion and early intervention are vital.

Ultraviolet exposure is the main risk factor; other factors include chronic immunosuppression (particularly in transplant recipients), infection with HPV, recurrent trauma and chronic scarring.

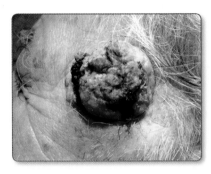

Figure 5.11 Squamous cell carcinoma.

Clinical features

The clinical presentation of SCC is very heterogeneous. Typically lesions present:

- as non-healing papules, crusted nodules (**Figure 5.11**) or verrucous forms which resemble a viral wart; they may also present as ulcerated skin
- on sun-exposed sites in older patients, such as the lips, pinna, scalp and lower legs
- on a background of photodamage and actinic change

Clinical insight

Keratoacanthoma is often referred to as an SCC, but it is an entity in its own right. It has no metastatic potential and the ability to regress. It presents as a rapidly growing nodule over a 6- to 9-week period, and it then undergoes rapid resolution.

Treatment

All patients with suspected SCC should be referred urgently to a specialist. A punch biopsy is taken to confirm the diagnosis. After this a number of treatment options are available, and the treatment decision is based on the histology, site and patient choice:

- surgical excision with a 4- to 6-mm margin (95% success rate)
- Mohs' micrographic surgery, considered when the lesion has a high-risk histological subtype, is located at a high risk site or is recurrent
- radiotherapy, which may be used for treatment or as an adjunct to surgery

5.5 Malignant melanoma

Malignant melanoma (**Figure 5.12**) accounts for only 4% of all skin cancers but it causes the greatest number of skin cancer-related deaths. It is a malignancy of the melanocytes. Melanomas can occur anywhere on the body; 50% arise from pre-existing moles and the rest are new lesions. The prognosis is based on the depth of invasion of the tumour, known as the Breslow thickness. There are a number of different subtypes of melanoma, as listed in **Table 5.6**.

Risk factors for melanoma include:
- UV light exposure
- family history (accounts for around 2%)
- dysplastic naevus syndrome (>50 atypical naevi increase risk fivefold)
- congenital naevus (giant congenital naevi >20 cm are more at risk)
- Fitzpatrick's skin phototype (type I signifies the greatest risk)

Clinical features

The **ABCDE criteria** (see **Table 5.7**) are a checklist that can be used for any suspicious pigmented lesion. The list comprises features that suggest malignancy. If all features are present the lesion is highly likely to be malignant. Dermatoscopy examination and

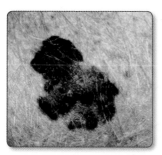

Figure 5.12 Superficial spreading malignant melanoma.

Subtype	Clinical features
Lentigo maligna melanoma	Found in elderly patients with background photodamage Found on the head and neck In situ component (lentigo maligna) can be present for years before becoming invasive Invasive nodules can be melanotic or amelanotic
Superficial spreading melanoma	Most common between 30 and 50 years of age Commonly found in sun-exposed sites (backs in men, lower legs in women)
Nodular melanoma	Seen in 15–30% of patients Most common on the legs or torso Grows rapidly over weeks or months
Acral lentiginous melanoma	Most common subtype in African–Caribbean patients Occurs on palmar plantar surfaces or the subungual area

Table 5.6 Subtypes of primary cutaneous melanoma and their clinical features

A	Asymmetrical lesion
B	Border irregularity: scalloped, 'plume of smoke' or notched border
C	Colour: more than two colours
D	Diameter >6 mm/dermatoscopic features
E	Evolving: changes in size, shape, colour

Table 5.7 Criteria to assess pigmented lesions

reflectance confocal microscopy can further help diagnosis and reduce the number of unnecessary biopsies.

Clinical insight

Sun protection advice should be given to all patients. In patients with very strict sun avoidance, vitamin D supplementation is recommended.

Treatment

Immediate referral should be made for an excision biopsy of the entire lesion; following diagnosis a second surgical procedure of wide local excision of 1–2 cm, depending on the Breslow thickness, is performed. A sentinel node biopsy may be offered to more accurately stage the melanoma, but offers no treatment benefit.

During follow-up it is important to examine for local or regional recurrence. Self-examination is also encouraged.

5.6 Rare skin cancers

Dermatofibromasarcoma protuberans

This is a rare malignant tumour arising in the deep dermis, it usually presents in early adult life, as a very slow-growing brown/red plaque or nodule on the skin (**Figure 5.13**). The lesion feels firm and rubbery and is often associated with subcutaneous spread, which may be palpable. Treatment is with Mohs' micrographic surgery due to its irregular growth pattern and high risk of local recurrence. DFSP rarely metastasises.

Merkel's cell cancer

This is a rare tumour arising from Merkel's cells, pressure receptors in the skin; it occurs in sun-exposed sites in elderly people. It can be very aggressive and metastasises, with a poor prognosis. It presents as a solitary red nodule, often

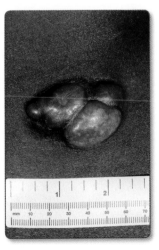

Figure 5.13 Dermatofibrosarcoma protuberans.

on the head and neck. Treatment is by surgical removal and radiotherapy.

Cutaneous T-cell lymphoma

This is a rare type of non-Hodgkin's lymphoma that affects the skin. Early stage disease clinically resembles eczema, as erythematous, dry patches on the skin. The most common types of cutaneous T-cell lymphoma are:

- **mycosis fungoides (MF):** erythematous patches, plaques and rarely nodules
- **Sézary's syndrome:** similar skin signs to MF but patients also have the same malignant T cells in the blood

Photodermatology

Photodermatology concerns diseases associated with ultraviolet radiation (UVR) and the use of UVR in the treatment of cutaneous disease.

The sun emits UVR of wavelengths between 200 nm and 400 nm (**Table 6.1**): the longer the wavelength, the deeper the penetration into the skin.

UVR exposure to the skin can cause:

- DNA damage leading to skin cancers
- activation of antigens, leading to 'photosensitive' eruptions
- photoageing through replacement of collagen with elastin
- local immunosuppressive and anti-inflammatory effects in the skin

Ultraviolet radiation is used in the treatment of a number of skin diseases (phototherapy).

Fitzpatrick's categorisation (**Table 6.2**) characterises skin types based on the propensity to tan or burn. There are multiple methods to prevent UV damage to the skin. Advice to patients should be as follows.

- **Avoidance**: sunlight has its greatest intensity between 10:00 and 16:00, so exposure should be reduced or avoided during these times.

> ## Clinical insight
>
> Photosensitive eruptions affect sun-exposed sites: face ears, 'V' area of neck and upper chest, and dorsal surface of forearms (**Figures 6.1** and **6.2**).
>
> Examine for sparing on 'shaded' areas: upper eyelids, nasolabial folds, cutaneous upper lip, under chin and posterior auricular skin.

UV radiation	Wavelength (nm)	Depth of penetration
UVA	400–320	Dermis
UVB	320–290	Epidermis
UVC	200–290	Absorbed by atmosphere

Table 6.1 Characteristics of ultraviolet (UV) radiation

Skin type	Colour	Characteristics
I	White	Always burns, never tans
II	White	Always burns, minimal tan
III	White–olive	Burns minimally, gradually tans
IV	Light brown	Burns minimally, tans well
V	Brown	Rarely burns, tans well
VI	Dark brown/black	Never burns, always tans

Table 6.2 Fitzpatrick's skin classification

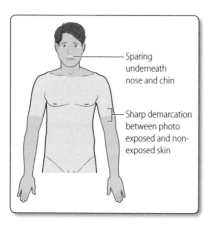

Figure 6.1 Distribution of photosensitive rash.

Sparing underneath nose and chin

Sharp demarcation between photo exposed and non-exposed skin

- **Protective clothing:** wear long sleeves, trousers and wide-brimmed hats.
- **Sunscreen:** this should be 'broad spectrum' (UVA and UVB) with a sun protection factor (SPF) ≥30 and applied 30 min before sun exposure and at 2-hourly intervals thereafter.

6.1 Clinical scenario

Presentation

A 24-year-old woman presents with an itchy rash affecting her face, back of hands and arms, and neck. It started 4 hours

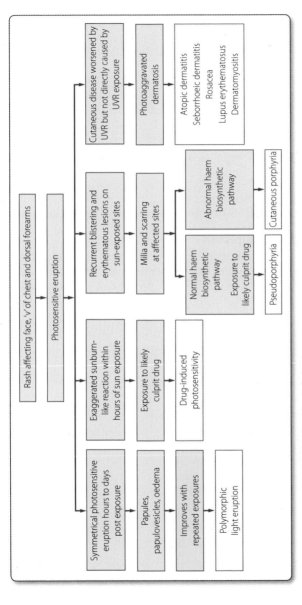

Figure 6.2 Diagnostic flowchart for photodistributed rash.

after sunbathing and has been present for 2 days. She recalls a few similar episodes after sun exposure. There is no history of blistering or any medication.

Diagnostic approach

The onset and distribution of the rash strongly suggest a photosensitive eruption. There is no obvious drug culprit. Any topical treatments, such as sun creams, should be considered as a cause of an irritant or allergic dermatitis. The main differentials are polymorphic light eruption and solar urticaria.

Examination

Grouped erythematous papules and evidence of excoriation are present on her face, arms and neck (see **Figure 6.3**).

Diagnostic approach

The diagnosis of polymorphic light eruption was made; however, conditions such as systemic lupus erythematosus (SLE) and porphyria should be excluded, therefore antinuclear

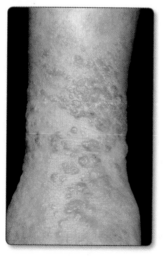

Figure 6.3 Polymorphic light eruption.

antibody (ANA), anti-Ro/SS-A and anti-La/SS-B tests, and/or measurement of porphyrin levels are required.

Management

Use of antihistamines may be helpful for pruritus. A 5-day course of a once-daily potent topical steroid is given and the patient advised about photoprotection.

6.2 Immunologically mediated photodermatoses

The most common example is polymorphic light eruption (PMLE). Less common examples include solar urticaria, actinic prurigo, hydrovacciniforme and chronic actinic dermatitis.

Polymorphic light eruption

A photosensitive eruption occurs hours to days after UVR exposure and is most severe in spring/early summer. It usually improves as summer goes on ('hardening').

Prevalence increases at increasing latitudes (1% in Singapore but 20% in Scandinavia). It occurs more commonly in women and those who are fair skinned. PMLE is a type IV contact hypersensitivity reaction to endogenous photo-induced cutaneous antigens.

Differential diagnoses include lupus erythematosus (LE), photoaggravated eczema and porphyria.

Clinical features

A symmetrical photosensitive eruption occurs hours to days after exposure to UVR.

The rash may consist of papulovesicles, vesicles, bullae or confluent oedematous plaques, and can last for several days.

Treatment

There are a number of options:
- Photoprotection, including broad-spectrum sunscreens, should be advised for all.

- A short course of a once-daily topical corticosteroid gives symptomatic relief.
- In patients with repeated annual episodes, phototherapy (narrow-band UVB or PUVA) may be given in early spring to induce tolerance and prevent eruptions later in the year. Oral corticosteroids may be used for acute PMLE.

6.3 Photosensitivity: exogenous agents

Agents applied to the skin or ingested can provoke a photosensitive rash when the individual is exposed to UVR.

Drug-induced photosensitivity

The drug or its metabolite triggers a rash in a photosensitive distribution on UV exposure.

Prevalence is estimated at 5%. The common culprits are doxycycline, non-steroidal anti-inflammatory drugs (NSAIDs), fluoroquinones and amiodarone.

Clinical features

Patients present with a painful, exaggerated, sunburn-like reaction in a photosensitive distribution which occurs *within hours of sun exposure.*

Treatment

Once the photosensitising agent has been withdrawn and the patient avoids UVR, the rash resolves with desquamation. A short course of topical steroids can be given for symptomatic relief.

Phytophotodermatitis

This is a phototoxic reaction in which a plant-derived photosensitising agent comes into direct contact with the skin. It is a delayed-type IV hypersensitivity reaction. An intense inflammatory reaction is provoked *around 24 hours after sun exposure.*

Individuals at risk of this are gardeners, hikers and those handling certain fruit and vegetables.

Clinical features

Patients present with painful erythema, oedema and blistering in a bizarre distribution. The last reflects the pattern of contact with the agent, e.g. linear erythema after contact with corn in a field, or over the thumb and dorsum of the hand after contact with the juice of limes.

> ### Clinical insight
>
> Common photosensitisers are limes, celery, parsnip, parsley, and other members of the Apiaceae and Rutaceae plant families.

Treatment

The condition is self-limiting, although it can leave significant post-inflammatory hyperpigmentation; this can take many months to resolve.

6.4 Cutaneous porphyrias and pseudoporphyria

Cutaneous porphyrias

The porphyrias are a set of genetic diseases caused by enzyme abnormalities in the haem biosynthetic pathways. They are associated with neurovisceral and cutaneous features. Porphyrins accumulate in the skin and are activated by UVR, leading to a photosensitive rash.

Clinical features

Patients present with recurrent blistering and erythematous lesions on sun-exposed sites. These can cause severe scarring and deformity, and can easily become infected. Age of presentation varies from childhood to the third or fourth decade.

Treatment

Photoprotection is advised for all patients. The treatment is for the underlying porphyria; it may include venesection, iron-chelating agents and hydroxychloroquine.

Pseudoporphyria

Pseudoprophyria is a photosensitive eruption that is associated with certain drugs, renal failure and sunbed use. The haem biosynthetic pathway is normal but the clinical features mimic a type of porphyria.

Differential diagnoses include bullous pemphigoid and bullous LE.

Clinical features

Bullae and vesicles appear on sun-exposed sites: the dorsum of the hands, forearms and face. Blisters heal with scarring and milia.

The most common drug culprits are NSAIDs, diuretics and retinoids. Even after cessation of the causative agent, the blistering rash can persist for many months.

Treatment

The culprit drug should be stopped immediately and the patient advised about photoprotection.

6.5 Photoexacerbated dermatoses

Some pre-existing skin diseases are exacerbated by exposure to UVR. Examples include LE (see page 188), dermatomyositis (see page 192) and atopic dermatitis (see page 126). Patients present with a flare of disease in a photosensitive distribution. Management is photoprotection and treatment of the underlying condition.

6.6 Phototherapy

This refers to the use of UVR to treat cutaneous disease. Conditions treated with phototherapy include psoriasis, atopic eczema, lichen planus, pruritus, vitiligo and cutaneous T-cell lymphoma. The two main types are UVB therapy and UVA plus psoralen (PUVA). Psoralen is a sensitiser that potentiates the effects of UVA on the skin.

Phototherapy is contraindicated in patients with xeroderma pigmentosum (XP, see page 249) or LE. It should be used with caution in patients with photosensitive disorders or a history of skin cancer, or who are immunosuppressed.

Patients are treated in walk-in cabinets with bulbs emitting UVR of a specific wavelength. Treatments are set to an appropriate level for the skin type, last for seconds initially and are increased as tolerated. A course comprises up to 30 treatments.

UVR is thought to improve skin disease through:

- local immunosuppression
- decreasing cell proliferation
- T-cell apoptosis

There are both long- and **short-term** side effects to phototherapy. In the short term patients may experience erythema (burning) and/or blistering, pruritus or recurrent cold sores (herpes simplex type 1 infection). The **long-term** effects include accelerated photoageing and an increased risk of skin cancer (more notable with UVA phototherapy).

Allergy

Allergy plays a role in many skin diseases. Certain skin diseases are exacerbated by hypersensitivity and others solely caused by hypersensitivity. The four main types of hypersensitivity reaction are:

1. Type I: immediate-type hypersensitivity, mediated by immunoglobulin (Ig) E molecules (see Figure 8.1)
2. Type II: antibody to cell-bound antigen
3. Type III: immune complex mediated
4. Type IV: delayed-type hypersensitivity mediated by T cells (see Figure 8.2)

Type I and IV reactions are the most relevant to allergy-mediated skin disease and allergy testing in dermatology.

Type I hypersensitivity reactions

These reactions occur within minutes and depend on antibodies. A well-known example is anaphylaxis, which occurs on first exposure to the antigen.

Exposure to or ingestion of exogenous antigen (e.g. drug metabolite, latex, bee venom) triggers the reaction. The antigen binds to IgE molecules on the surface of mast cells and basophils. This leads to breakdown or 'degranulation' of the mast cells. Within minutes a weal-and-flare response occurs and the skin quickly becomes red and swollen. In serious cases swelling also occurs in the airways, leading to obstruction and respiratory arrest.

Type IV hypersensitivity reactions

These reactions occur over days and in some over weeks; they are mediated by T cells (i.e. antibody independent). On first exposure to the antigen, no reaction occurs but, as a result of the exposure, T cells are produced to the antigen. This is known as sensitisation. At the next exposure to the antigen, these T cells are activated. As a consequence a number of cytokines are released, leading to skin inflammation. The time from antigen exposure to skin inflammation may be days or even weeks in some cases.

7.1 Clinical scenario

A 27-year-old woman presents with a 3-month history of a persistent bilateral periorbital rash (**Figure 7.1**). It is itchy and scaly, and lasts for weeks at a time. There is no history of malaise, change in vision or rash anywhere else. She had eczema as a child and does not take any medications regularly. The patient is a journalist for a fashion magazine.

On examination the patient is wearing make-up, including mascara and eyeliner. On removal of these there is a bilateral, eczematous, intensely erythematous eruption on her eyelids. There is no skin disease elsewhere.

Diagnostic approach

Symmetrical eyelid dermatitis, without evidence of eczema elsewhere, suggests that this may be secondary to an exogenous agent around the eyes causing a dermatitis.

The patient uses cosmetic products and these may contain chemicals that can trigger allergic contact dermatitis (ACD). In cases of eyelid eczema, it is also important to ask patients if they use nail varnish (the patient can rub their eyes, leading to ACD) and eyelash curlers, because these usually contain nickel, which can trigger ACD.

Investigations

Patch testing is performed to the European Standard Battery (see page 109); this confirms an ACD to methylisothiazolinone, a preservative commonly used in cosmetic products.

Diagnostic approach

The patient is asked to review all the products that she uses

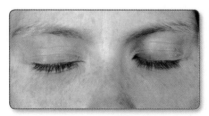

Figure 7.1 Eyelid dermatitis.

on the eye area that may contain methylisothiazolinone. The patient finds that it is in her cleansing wipes and her mascara. She is counselled to avoid all products containing methylisothiazolinone; acute treatment with 1% hydrocortisone ointment for 7 days leads to resolution of the rash.

7.2 Allergic contact dermatitis

Allergic contact dermatitis occurs with low-molecular-weight antigens (<1 kDa) that bind to skin proteins, known as haptens. Haptens are presented to T lymphocytes and a memory population of T cells is made. Re-exposure to the relevant hapten leads to migration of effector T cells to the skin, with subsequent release of inflammatory mediators and development of a rash.

Allergic contact dematitis is a common cause of occupational dermatosis. Workers at high risk of developing this allergy include hairdressers, beauticians, healthcare workers and construction workers. Common culprits are latex materials, cleansers, resins and acrylics.

> **Clinical insight**
>
> Before patch testing, it is crucial to take a detailed history of the patient's occupation, hobbies, and any cosmetic or household products used.

In recent years there has been an epidemic of ACD secondary to the preservative methylisothiazolinone, which is used in many cosmetic and household products. The incidence of ACD increases with age, which reflects increasing exposure

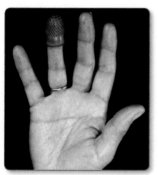

Figure 7.2 Allergic contact dermatitis of the fingers to rubber.

and sensitisation to haptens with age. ACD is also common in patients with atopic dermatitis and chronic actinic dermatitis.

Clinical features

Clinical features of ACD include:

- erythematous, scaly, eczematous plaques in the distribution of the contact with the allergen (**Figure 7.2**)
- vesicles or bullae in severe cases
- oedematous, confluent erythema in affected areas; in hair dye allergy, patient may present with marked periorbital oedema

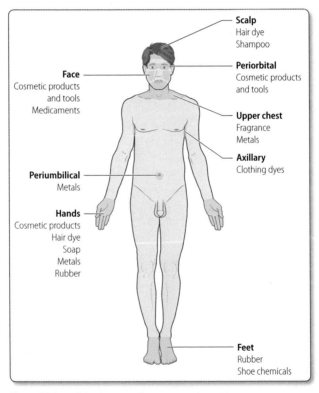

Scalp
Hair dye
Shampoo

Periorbital
Cosmetic products
and tools

Face
Cosmetic products
and tools
Medicaments

Upper chest
Fragrance
Metals

Axillary
Clothing dyes

Periumbilical
Metals

Hands
Cosmetic products
Hair dye
Soap
Metals
Rubber

Feet
Rubber
Shoe chemicals

Figure 7.3 Sites of distribution in allergic contact dermatitis.

Typically these features are present at the site of exposure to the allergen, e.g. on the scalp and ears in hair dye allergy; classic distribution sites are shown in **Figure 7.3**.

Treatment

The patient should have patch testing performed to the European Standard Battery and any other relevant series of allergens. If a positive allergen is noted, the patient should avoid contact with the substance to see whether this relieves symptoms. For acute disease, depending on the severity, the patient can be treated with an emollient and potent topical corticosteroid ointment (mild strength in the periorbital area).

7.3 Prick testing

Prick testing is used to detect type I hypersensitivity reactions and the presence of allergen-specific IgE molecules on the surface of mast cells. It is also used to detect allergies to food, venom, airborne agents and latex.

Prick testing is contraindicated in patients who have recently had anaphylaxis or a high risk of anaphylaxis with an allergen. Patients with the following conditions cannot have skin testing because activation of their underlying disease leads to false-positive results: acute or chronic urticaria and cutaneous mastocytosis.

Generally it is recommended that patients stop antihistamines 3–5 days before testing. If possible prednisolone should also be stopped 3 days before testing.

Method

- Commercial solutions containing a low concentration of allergen are used.
- The volar aspect of the forearm is used and the skin is cleansed before testing.
- A droplet of allergen solution is placed on skin (**Figure 7.4**).
- A commercially available test device is used to prick through the droplets of allergen.
- A positive control (histamine) and a negative control (saline) are used, and introduced into the skin as outlined above.

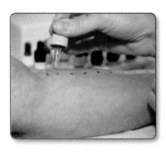

Figure 7.4 Prick testing.

Clinical insight

Prick testing identifies allergens in type I hypersensitivity reactions. It should not be used if there is a history of anaphylaxis to an allergen.

The results are read after 15 minutes. A positive reaction is defined as a weal that is equal in size to or larger than the histamine reaction. A positive reaction indicates the presence of IgE molecules only to the allergen in question. In order to be labelled 'allergic' the patient must have a history of reaction on exposure to the allergen.

A negative result predicts the absence of an IgE reaction with 95% accuracy.

7.4 Patch testing

This is used to detect type IV hypersensitivity reactions. Patients have already been sensitised to the allergen and repeated exposure to a controlled concentration recreates a delayed-type hypersensitivity reaction.

Indications for patch testing include:
- history and eczematous rash suggestive of ACD
- chronic dermatitis of eyelids, face, hands or feet
- eczema in patients who work in high-risk occupations (e.g. healthcare workers, hairdressers)
- patients with atopic dermatitis in whom ACD is a suspected exacerbating factor

History taking

This is one of the most important steps in ensuring that the correct allergens are identified. It is similar to detective work, trying to identify all aspects of the patient's life and habits that could be leading to contact with an allergen. This must include a full history of the dermatitis (onset, morphology, distribution, exacerbations and previous treatments). The patient's occupation (details of work environment) and social history, including hobbies and cosmetic 'habits', e.g. hair dyes, eyelash curler use, are also important.

Selection of allergen

An internationally agreed 'standard' series of the most common contact allergens are tested for in most cases. Additional series (e.g. fragrance series, hairdresser series) contain a larger number of potential allergens and are available if required. The need for these more detailed tests should be determined according to the patient's history and clinical signs, and the suspected culprit allergen. Examples of potential allergens tested as part of the European Standard Battery Series are found in **Table 7.1**.

Patients may also be tested with their own cosmetic products and drugs. Patch testing to detect drug allergy has a low sensitivity (i.e. a negative result does not exclude allergy to the drug in question).

Allergens are purchased in commercially available preparations, usually using petroleum jelly.

Substance	Example
Metals	Nickel sulphate, potassium dichromate
Rubber additives	Thiuram mix, carba mix
Hair dye	*p*-Phenylenediamine
Cosmetic preservatives	Methylisothiazolinone, sodium metabisulphite

Table 7.1 Examples of substances in the European Standard Battery series

Method of patch testing

Patch testing is a time-consuming process that requires at least three visits during a specified week. Testing is usually performed on the back. Disease activity on the back has to be low because application of tests can lead to exacerbation of any underlying skin condition. Patients should be advised to avoid getting the test area wet through showering/bathing, excessive sweating and warm environments.

Each allergen is placed in a separate 'chamber' and all the chambers are applied to the patient's skin, usually on the back (**Figure 7.5**). These stay in place for 2 days before the first readings are taken. Departments vary in practice but in most cases a further reading is taken 2 days later.

Prednisolone at a dose of up to 10 mg can be continued during patch testing. Patients should be advised not to apply topical corticosteroids to their backs during testing. Oral antihistamines do not need to be stopped.

Interpretation

The International Contact Dermatitis Research Group has developed a scoring system for evaluating patch test reactions (**Table 7.2**).

Any reactions identified have to be interpreted in terms of clinical relevance. The allergy may or may not be relevant to the

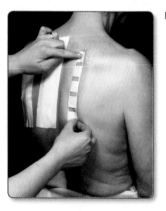

Figure 7.5 Patch testing.

Score	Interpretation
−	Negative reaction
?/+	Doubtful reaction: faint erythema
+	Weak reaction: erythema, slight infiltration
++	Strong reaction: erythema, infiltration, vesicles
+++	Extreme reaction: bullous, ulcerative
IR	Irritant reactions
NT	Not tested

Table 7.2 International Contact Dermatitis Research Group score

patient's current problem, e.g. an allergy to a thiuram mix in the patient in the clinical scenario above would not be relevant to her current problem, but an allergy to methylisothiazolinone would be.

In cases of occupational dermatitis, it may be necessary to visit the work environment ('site visit') to identify potential allergens. When an allergen is identified patients should be advised to avoid it to minimise their symptoms.

7.5 Atopy

This is the genetic tendency to produce IgE antibodies when exposed to an allergen. Atopic dermatitis, allergic rhinitis (hay fever) and asthma are thought to occur because of this tendency. Indeed, 80% of children with atopic dermatitis go on to develop allergic rhinitis and/or asthma (so-called atopic march).

7.6 Food allergy, aeroallergens and eczema

Food allergy can play a role in eczema in some children but it is rare for it to do so in adults.

Around 30% of children with severe eczema are thought to have a food allergy contributing to their skin disease. These children tend to have elevated serum IgE levels compared with children with milder eczema. The most common food allergen identified on prick testing is egg. Food should be omitted from the diet only if there is sufficient clinical suspicion and evidence of allergy on testing, as well as evidence of improvement on removal of the allergen from the diet.

Common aeroallergens that exacerbate atopic dermatitis are house-dust mite, cat or dog dander, and grass pollen. These can all exacerbate disease, so affected patients should be advised to avoid them where possible.

Drug reactions

Cutaneous drug reactions are common, with an estimated 10 cases per 1000 new users of a drug (**Table 8.1**). An accurate drug history is essential to identify the culprit.

Most reactions are not life threatening, although there is a subset of severe cutaneous adverse reactions (SCARs) that have a significant morbidity and mortality.

Drug reactions are hypersensitivity reactions and can be either type I (immediate – **Figure 8.1**) or type IV (delayed – **Figure 8.2**). Immediate reactions are mediated by IgE and occur within minutes of exposure, as seen in anaphylaxis. Delayed reactions are mediated by T cells and take days or weeks to evolve.

Clinical insight

Always obtain an accurate drug history and do not forget about 'over-the-counter' medications from pharmacies or supermarkets.

Clinical insight

Establish a clear timeline between onset of rash and medications taken, to help identify the drug that is the most likely culprit.

8.1 Clinical scenario

Itchy rash

Presentation

A 46-year-old woman with a diagnosis of seronegative arthritis was started on sulfasalazine. Six weeks later she presents to hospital with facial swelling, malaise, a fever of 39°C and a 3-day history of an itchy rash.

Diagnostic approach

The malaise, fever and rash mean that an infectious cause for this presentation must be investigated. Sulfasalazine is known to cause drug rashes, so a systemic reaction to a drug must be considered.

Drug reaction	Likely causative agent	Time between drug exposure and onset of rash
Drug-induced exanthem	Penicillins Cepahlosporins Sulfonamides Carbamazepine Phenytoin	2 weeks (sooner on re-exposure)
Urticaria and angio-oedema	Penicillins Cephalosporins Sulfonamides Opiates Aspirin Non-steroidal anti-inflammatory drugs (NSAIDs) Vancomycin Angiotensin-converting enzyme inhibitors	May occur within minutes, hours or days
Stevens–Johnson syndrome/ toxic epidermal necrolysis	Allopurinol Sulfonamides NSAIDs Phenytoin Carbamazepine	1–3 weeks
Acute generalised exanthematous pustulosis	Penicillin Macrolides Calcium channel blockers Antimalarial agents	1–3 days
Drug hypersensitivity syndrome	Allopurinol Penicillin Phenytoin Carbamazepine	2–6 weeks
Erythema multiforme	Herpes simplex virus Mycoplasma pneumoniae Sulfonamides NSAIDs	0–3 weeks
Fixed drug eruption	Penicillins Sulfonamides Tetracyclines NSAIDs Paracetamol Antimalarial agents	14 days (within 24 hours on re-exposure to drug)

Table 8.1 Cutaneous drug reactions.

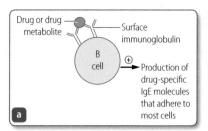

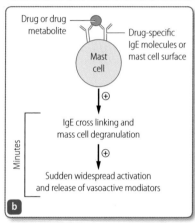

Figure 8.1 Type 1 hypersensitivity reaction: (a) stage 1: sensitisation – onset is immediate and regulated by IgE. (b) Re-exposure and reaction within minutes. The reactions are mediated by IgE and have an immediate onset (within minutes). Examples include anaphylaxis and angio-oedema.

Examination and investigations

On examination, there is marked facial oedema with associated subcorneal pustulation, jaundiced sclerae, and cervical and axillary lymphadenopathy. There is a widespread morbilliform erythema, which is confluent in places. Dusky, targetoid lesions are seen on the lower limbs (**Figure 8.3**). Investigation results are listed in **Table 8.2**.

Diagnostic approach

The key clinical features are:
- exposure to sulfasalazine
- facial swelling
- heterogeneous rash
- widespread lymphadenopathy

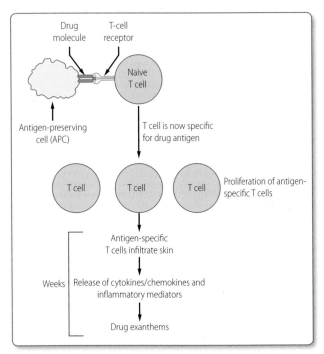

Figure 8.2 Type IV hypersensitivity reaction: these are mediated by T cells and have a delayed onset (within weeks). Examples include drug exanthems.

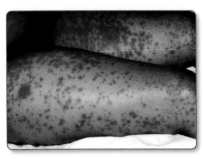

Figure 8.3 Drug hypersensitivity reaction.

Investigation	Result
Full blood count	Eosinophilia, lymphopaenia, atypical lymphocytes on blood film
Liver function tests	Transaminitis and bilirubin
Hepatitis screen, EBV/CMV serology/HIV	All negative
Full septic screen	Negative
Radiology: CT of the chest/abdomen/pelvis	Large para-aortic and gastric lymph nodes
CMV, cytomegalovirus; CT, computerised tomography; EBV, Epstein–Barr virus; HIV, human immunodeficiency virus	

Table 8.2 Investigation results

- pyrexia
- eosinophilia
- abnormal liver function tests

These features are classic for the drug hypersensitivity syndrome (DHS) and a latency (time from drug exposure to cutaneous features) of 6 weeks is typical. DHS occurs because of an accentuated immune response to components of the culprit drug, leading to systemic inflammation.

It is crucial to ensure that a full septic screen is performed because sepsis is a key differential to exclude. When DHS is diagnosed:

- the culprit drug (in this case sulfasalazine) is stopped immediately
- potent topical steroids are prescribed to help treat the associated rash
- systemic steroids (oral or intravenous) are required to control the systemic features (fever, deranged blood count and liver function tests)

8.2 Drug-induced exanthems

Ninety per cent of drug induced rashes are exanthems; they present within 2 weeks of starting a new medication. If there has been previous exposure (i.e. sensitisation), the rash may start within a couple of days.

Drug exanthems are called morbilliform because they resemble the clinical appearance of measles (**Figure 8.4**). Viruses (including HIV) can cause a similar rash and should be considered as differentials to a drug exanthems.

Clinical features

Patients develop a symmetrical, macular, erythematous rash which blanches on pressure. The rash is pruritic and may extend from the initial site to involve multiple areas of the body. It is often associated with a low-grade fever (<38.5°C).

Drug exanthems evolve rapidly and resolve within about a week of cessation of the drug. Patients should be advised to avoid the culprit drug because it may cause a more severe reaction on re-exposure.

Treatment

Management is by prompt identification and withdrawal of the suspected culprit drug, and supportive care. Pruritus is treated with sedating antihistamines, potent topical steroids and emollients.

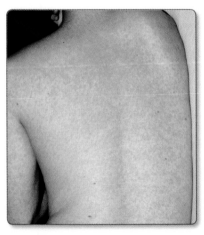

Figure 8.4 Drug-induced exanthem.

8.3 Urticaria

Urticaria (hives or nettle rash) accounts for 5% of all drug reactions (**Figure 8.5**). It manifests as a transient superficial erythema and oedema in the skin. Differential diagnoses to consider are other causes of urticaria (infection, vasculitis, idiopathic) and erythema multiforme.

Angio-oedema is a related condition that may be triggered by medication. It can lead to airway obstruction (see page 269).

Clinical features

Patients develop pruritic, well-circumscribed plaques with central pallor. These weals can occur at multiple sites, anywhere on the body. They are usually transient, lasting under 24 hours. Urticaria can occur within minutes of exposure or may take hours or days to evolve.

Treatment

The suspected causative agent should be withdrawn as soon as possible, and non-sedating antihistamines started. In severe cases oral steroids may be needed.

Clinical insight

Apparently uncomplicated drug reactions can evolve into more serious SCAR syndromes and should be monitored carefully.

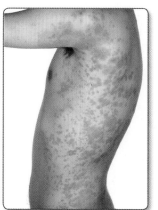

Figure 8.5 Urticaria.

8.4 Severe cutaneous adverse reactions

Stevens–Johnson syndrome and toxic epidermal necrolysis

See page 275.

Acute generalised exanthematous pustulosis

Acute generalised exanthematous pustulosis (AGEP) has an incidence of 1–5/million per year.

Patients with AGEP present with widespread monomorphic pustules and skin swelling (**Figure 8.6**). These start between 1 and 3 days after exposure – this short period suggests previous exposure to the culprit drug. Differential diagnoses include acute pustular psoriasis and angio-oedema.

Clinical features

Patients present:
- with swelling and itchy erythema in the flexures and on the face

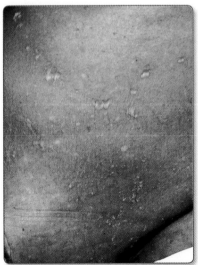

Figure 8.6 Acute generalised exanthematous pustulosis.

- with sheets of widespread monomorphic pustules, fever (>38°C), tachycardia and an elevated neutrophil count

Treatment

The culprit agent should be stopped immediately. Emollients and potent topical steroid therapy should be introduced and fluid losses replaced intravenously if required. Moist dressings and an antibacterial wash can be used when pustules are present. Resolution occurs within 5–7 days.

Drug hypersensitivity syndrome

Drug hypersensitivity syndrome (or drug reaction with eosinophilia and systemic symptoms) is a severe cutaneous reaction to medication that can be life threatening, and usually presents 2–6 weeks after exposure. Its incidence is estimated at 9 per million per year.

Differential diagnoses include other SCAR syndromes, e.g. Stevens–Johnson syndrome, toxic epidermal necrolysis (TEN), AGEP, acute lupus erythematosus and T-cell lymphoma.

Clinical features

Patients present with:
- widespread maculopapular or morbilliform erythema with cutaneous oedema, often marked around the face and ears
- fever (>38°C), tachycardia and hypotension
- lymphadenopathy at multiple sites (e.g. cervical, axillary, inguinal)
- deranged liver function tests
- eosinophilia and atypical lymphocytes

Treatment

Any suspected culprit drug should be withdrawn, and potent topical steroids and emollients initiated immediately. Oral or intravenous prednisolone is required to treat systemic features. Despite withdrawal of the causative agent, the reaction can last for months and the patient's liver function should continue to be monitored.

8.5 Fixed drug eruption

Fixed drug eruptions (FDEs) account for 2–3% of drug reactions. They typically comprise a single or small number of well-circumscribed erythematous plaques. Key differentials include:

- single lesions: an arthropod bite
- multiple lesions and mucosal involvement: erythema multiforme or Stevens–Johnson syndrome

Clinical features

Patients present with a well-demarcated erythematous or violaceous plaque, most often on the hands, feet, genitals or face. The plaque may erode or blister, or be pruritic or described as burning or stinging.

Lesions occur up to 14 days after first exposure to the drug, and within 24 hours at identical sites on re-exposure.

The lesions appear over the course of hours and fade over the course of several days, often leaving post-inflammatory hyperpigmentation.

Treatment

The likely causative agent should be withdrawn as soon as possible. Moderately potent topical steroids can be used for 7–10 days, along with oral, non-sedating antihistamines.

8.6 Erythema multiforme

This is most commonly caused by infection (see page 166).

Inflammatory dermatology

Inflammatory dermatology denotes the involvement of the inflammatory response in the pathogenesis of a skin disease. Clinically it is characterised by erythema, pain, swelling and heat. Inflammation can occur without infection, an important point to note because the two are often confused. Common inflammatory conditions include eczema, psoriasis, bullous pemphigoid and venous eczema. Treatment is focused on control of disease rather than cure.

9.1 Clinical scenario

Presentation

A 72-year-old man presents to the accident and emergency department with bilateral leg pain and swelling. His lower legs have become red and started weeping over the past month. Before that they had been quite dry and itchy. His past medical history includes hypertension, for which he takes a calcium channel blocker; he also had his varicose veins stripped 4 years ago. He lives alone. There is no history of dyspnoea.

Diagnostic approach

The patient's age, history of dry skin and varicose veins suggest venous insufficiency and stasis eczema. An important point is that this is **bilateral** disease; the main differential diagnosis for an acute red leg would be cellulitis, which is usually a **unilateral** disease (**Figure 9.1**).

It is imperative to assess whether the patient has any signs of heart failure, especially if presenting with bilateral swollen legs.

Examination and investigations

He is afebrile with normal oxygen saturations and heart rate, and a blood pressure of 150/95 mmHg. There is bilateral oedema distal to the mid-calf and a confluent, scaly erythema on both lower legs, with a sloughy discharge and crusting in

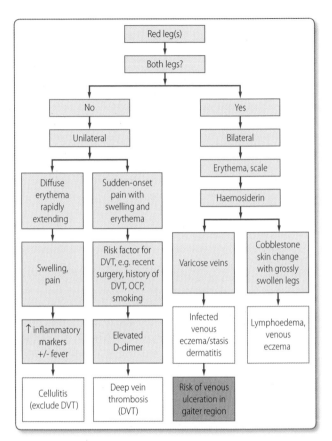

Figure 9.1 Diagnostic flowchart – the red leg.
OCP, oral contraceptive pill.

places. Brown pigment deposits around the ankles are noted and the skin around the ankles is firm. There are varicose veins on his right leg. Jugular venous pressure (JVP) is not elevated and his chest is clear on auscultation.

Bloods show a normal white cell count with a mild elevation of the C-reactive protein (CRP) at 18 mg/L. Swabs are sent from the sloughy areas.

Diagnostic approach
Key clinical features
The following are the key clinical features (**Figure 9.1**).

- **Bilateral leg oedema and erythema to mid-calf:** cellulitis and deep vein thrombosis (DVT) are almost always unilateral processes and should not be considered initially.
- **Normal JVP and no chest signs on auscultation**: no evidence of heart failure.
- **Varicose veins in right leg:** patient has venous reflux and insufficiency, which has led to dependent oedema to the calf.
- **Brown pigment deposits around ankles:** capillaries in the dermis become damaged due to oedema and venous reflux. Red blood cells leak from the capillaries and degrade, leaving haemosiderin, a brown pigment.
- **Indurated skin at the ankles:** this is scar tissue secondary to chronic venous insufficiency and is a lipodermatosclerosis.
- **Scaly erythema on both lower legs with sloughy discharge and crusting:** stasis eczema is an inflammatory process that typically presents with these signs and is associated with venous insufficiency.

Treatment
Treatment was started that was appropriate for infected venous eczema.

> **Clinical insight**
>
> Leg cellulitis is a unilateral disease, and stasis eczema a bilateral one.

9.2 Eczema

'Eczema' and 'dermatitis' are interchangeable terms for skin disease characterised by diffuse, itchy, erythematous, scaly eruptions. It is not a diagnosis in itself. Different subtypes of eczema with different causes are discussed below. All subtypes are chronic disease that may recur at any time, and physicians aim to control rather than cure them. This is an important message to give to patients. Treatment plans should be explained thoroughly and

> **Clinical insight**
>
> If it does not itch it is unlikely to be eczema.

clearly, be written down for them and be suitable to fit in with their lifestyles and capabilities.

An explanation of topical therapies and their application is detailed in Chapter 3.

Atopic dermatitis

The term 'atopy' refers to the genetic predisposition to produce immunoglobulin (Ig) E after exposure to allergens. Immune responses to allergens, irritants and microbes are all thought to play a role in atopic dermatitis. In certain cases aeroallergens (e.g. grass pollen) and food allergens (e.g. egg) trigger atopic dermatitis. Patients more commonly have other 'atopic' diseases such as asthma or hay fever. Genes (e.g. *FLG*, gene for filaggrin) involved in epidermal barrier function and hydration are defective in many patients with atopic dermatitis, so appropriate use of emollients is imperative in treating the disease.

Atopic dermatitis is very common and usually presents in childhood before the age of 5 years. It occurs in 15–20% of all schoolchildren in the UK. Environmental irritants may exacerbate atopic dermatitis, including bubble bath products, soaps, inhaled allergens and *Staphylococcus aureus*. Dietary factors aggravate atopic dermatitis in 10% of children, less commonly in adults. Endogenous factors such as stress can lead to flares of disease.

Important differential diagnoses include contact dermatitis, seborrhoeic dermatitis, drug reactions and scabies.

Diagnostic criteria

The patient must have itchy skin PLUS three or more of the following:
- itchiness at flexural skin creases
- history of asthma or hay fever
- dry skin in the past year
- visible flexural eczema (or affecting the cheeks/forehead/outer limbs in child aged <4 years)

Clinical features

The patient will generally have **dry** skin with **itchy, red**, scaly lesions on the **flexural** surfaces (**Figure 9.2**). In infants, the

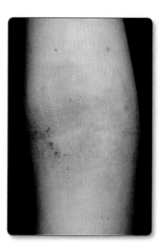

Figure 9.2 Atopic dermatitis.

cheeks, extensor surfaces and scalp are usually the first sites to be noticed as having erythematous scaly lesions. Due to chronic scratching the skin may become **lichenified**; the creases on the skin appear more pronounced as the skin thickens.

As a result of the defective barrier of the skin in atopic dermatitis, there is a higher incidence of infection. Bacterial infection is suggested when lesions become golden and crusted and have surrounding erythema, and there is a flare of the underlying disease. Eczema-infected herpes simplex virus is termed 'eczema herpeticum'; it is suggested by areas of rapidly worsening eczema, usually on the face – clustered pinched-out erosions. Such patients usually have marked fever and need to be dealt with as an emergency.

Patients may also present with erythroderma.

Treatment

Detailed application and the appropriate agents are discussed in Chapter 3.

Emollients These are used to create a barrier and hydrate the skin. These can be very greasy petroleum-based ointments or lighter creams. They should be used frequently and as regular baseline treatment in **all** cases.

Topical agents These suppress the immune system locally and include the following:

- **Topical corticosteroids:** these range in potency from weak (1% hydrocortisone) to superpotent (clobetasol propionate), depending on the body site and severity of disease (**Table 9.1**). This is the first-line treatment for all patients.
- **Topical calcineurin inhibitors:** these are a very useful alternative to topical steroids and roughly equivalent to low-potency topical steroids. The 0.1% tacrolimus preparation should be used in adults and the 0.03% preparation in children. They are particularly useful on the face and neck, and in skinfolds. Patients may report burning or stinging but otherwise they are generally very well tolerated.

> ### Clinical insight
>
> Topical calcineurin inhibitors should *not* be used when concomitant infection is suspected; they should be used just as maintenance therapy.

Some patients respond well to **TL0-1 phototherapy** (see page 100), which should be considered in patients who wish to try an alternative to topical steroid therapy.

Systemic agents These can be used in more severe cases of eczema and should be initiated by a dermatologist. Monitoring of blood tests can be shared between the dermatologist and the general practitioner.

Potency	Corticosteroid	Examples of proprietary names
Super potent (600 times as potent as hydrocortisone)	Clobetasol propionate Betamethasone dipropionate	Dermovate Diprosone
Potent (100–150 times as potent as hydrocortisone)	Mometasone furoate Betamethasone valerate	Elocon Betnovate
Moderate (2–25 times as potent as hydrocortisone)	Clobetasone butyrate	Eumovate
Mild	Hydrocortisone	Hydrocortisone
Fingertip unit: the amount of ointment/cream squeezed out of its tube from the end of the finger to the most distal crease on the index finger.		

Table 9.1 Steroid potency and fingertip unit

Commonly used agents are ciclosporin, azathioprine, mycophenolate mofetil and methotrexate. There is extensive work in the development of **biologic agents** to treat eczema effectively.

Seborrhoeic dermatitis

This occurs in 1–5% of the population, in both infants and adults, with a peak incidence in adolescence. It occurs in skin rich in sebaceous glands and is associated with an inflammatory reaction to the yeast *Malassezia*. Patients with HIV or Parkinson's disease are more likely to have this condition and symptoms may be made worse by illness, stress and immunosuppression. Differential diagnoses include psoriasis and rosacea.

Clinical features

Clinical features of seborrhoeic dermatitis include:
- discrete erythematous plaques with greasy yellowish scales in a distinct distribution over the nasolabial folds, bridge of nose, glabellar area or behind the ears
- dandruff – desquamation with any rash
  Seborrhoeic dermatitis may:
- affect the upper trunk, axillae and groin
- be more widespread in patients with HIV

Treatment

Scalp treatment to control dandruff is a shampoo containing 2% ketoconazole; it should applied to the scalp for 5–10 min three times a week until clear. This should be followed by regular use of selenium sulphide shampoo. To reduce itching, a potent steroid shampoo or foam should be used once weekly for 2–4 weeks.

Advice for the face and trunk is to avoid soap, to use 2% ketoconazole shampoo as a wash to the skin, and to use 1% hydrocortisone ointment in combination with an anti-fungal for 2 weeks to control symptoms. For eyelid disease, diluted baby shampoo applied with a cotton bud may be helpful.

> **Clinical insight**
>
> In patients presenting with widespread seborrhoeic dermatitis, a diagnosis of HIV should be considered.

More severe disease may require oral antifungal medication or UVB phototherapy.

Stasis dermatitis

Also known as varicose eczema or gravitational eczema (see Chapter 3), this is a common inflammatory rash on the legs associated with venous insufficiency. Dysfunction of venous valves leads to decreased venous return and increased pressure in the perforating vessels of the venous system – so-called venous hypertension. This insufficiency in the venous system leads to fluid leakage from capillaries, causing oedema and eczematous change. Its prevalence and its associated morbidity occur in about 3% of the population. Risk factors include older age, increased body mass index (BMI), previous DVT and an occupation that involves a lot of standing and/or walking.

Clinical features

Patients present with **bilateral** inflammatory leg eczema. The typical distribution is around the ankles (gaiter region) but it can extend proximally to the knee.

Patients present with a mix of characteristic features (**Figure 9.3**), for example:

- varicose veins – more evident when the patient stands
- widespread erythematous skin change with scaling or crusting
- brown macular areas on the skin – haemosiderin deposits
- lipodermatosclerosis – hardened, tight skin on the inner calf

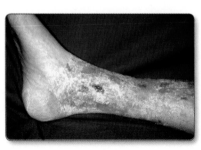

Figure 9.3 Venous eczema.

- atrophie blanche – porcelain-white, star-shaped scarring
- ulcers in the gaiter region
- secondary lymphoedema

Treatment

For all patients the aim is to control the venous hypertension in the legs. Arterial–brachial pressure index (ABPI) measurements should be performed to exclude significant peripheral arterial disease and then use:

- below-knee compression hosiery (see Chapter 3)
- leg elevation, exercise, weight reduction
- basic skin care with regular emollient use

If the skin is very inflamed, use moderate or potent topical steroid therapy according to severity of disease. If there is crusting soaks such as potassium permanganate or copper sulphate may be used.

It is essential to give the patient a thorough explanation that this is a chronic disease, plus the fact that it will take a long time to heal. Poor compliance with compression hosiery will worsen the prognosis.

Complications

Complications include:

> **Clinical insight**
>
> Leg compression hosiery is contraindicated in patients with significant peripheral arterial disease.

- allergic contact dermatitis, which can occur in reaction to the compression hosiery or topical therapies used to treat inflammation
- venous ulceration

Allergic contact dermatitis

See page 105.

Irritant contact dermatitis

This is a localised eczema that occurs due to exposure to chemical or physical agents. It is the most common cause of hand eczema and a very common cause of occupational eczema, e.g. in healthcare workers, food handlers, cleaners and hairdressers.

Examples of chemical irritants include water, detergents, oxidising agents such as bleach, and alkaline agents such as soap, cement and chalk. Physical irritants include metals, woods, plants and cold temperatures. Exposure to agents leads to disruption of the epidermal barrier, cytotoxic effects on keratinocytes and subsequent inflammation.

Differential diagnoses include allergic contact dermatitis (ACD), atopic dermatitis, hand eczema and scabies infection. Patch testing (see page 108) is required to exclude ACD.

Clinical features

A thorough history is required to make the diagnosis of irritant contact dermatitis (ICD). The patient's daily activities should be discussed, including hand hygiene routine, workplace environment and hobbies. Patients may be able to correlate the signs and symptoms with a particular activity. If it is associated with their occupation it is likely to improve at weekends and during holidays.

Patients give a history of:
- new onset or worsening of hand eczema
- painful, burning sensation in affected areas
- pruritus

Signs include localised eczematous change (e.g. hands only) with extensive erythema, scaling and fissuring (**Figure 9.4**).

It is vital to perform a full skin check to exclude the differential diagnoses for ICD.

Treatment

Identification of the irritant and minimisation of irritant exposure are a key part of treatment. In all cases regular use of

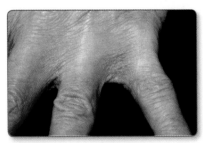

Figure 9.4 Irritant contact dermatitis.

emollients and gentle antimicrobial washes is recommended. Topical corticosteroid therapy may also be used to get severe disease under control.

Lichen simplex chronicus and nodular prurigo

These conditions are associated with chronic pruritus. Scratching and rubbing lead to inflammation in the skin and prompt further itching or rubbing; this is known as the itch–scratch cycle.

Adults, who may or may not have pre-existing skin disease, are most commonly affected. Patients should be examined for signs of conditions such as stasis dermatitis or atopic dermatitis which

> ### Clinical insight
>
> A full pruritic screen to exclude systemic causes of itch should be performed (renal function, thyroid function, liver function, full blood count, LDH, HIV test).

may be a trigger for pruritus. They should also be screened for evidence of anxiety and obsessive–compulsive disorder (see Chapter 16).

Renal disease, cholestasis, thyroid disease, HIV and lymphoproliferative disorders may all cause chronic pruritus.

Clinical features

Lichen simplex chronicus (Figure 9.5) In this condition the following features will be seen.
- The skin looks thickened and 'leathery' with exaggerated skin lines
- The affected skin may be hyperpigmented
- The most commonly affected sites are neck, scalp, lower legs, forearms and genital area

Nodular prurigo This shows the following:
- firm, dome-shaped itchy nodules

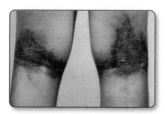

Figure 9.5 Lichen simplex chronicus.

- common sites of involvement: the arms, legs and upper back, i.e. areas within the patient's reach

Treatment

The aims of treatment are to break the itch–scratch cycle and reduce skin inflammation. Some or all of the following may be useful:

- topical corticosteroids under occlusion
- intralesional steroid into focal areas
- regular antihistamines
- emollients containing menthol
- cognitive–behavioural therapy and selective serotonin reuptake inhibitors which may be useful in certain cases

9.3 Papulosquamous skin disease

These disorders have prominent erythema and thick scaling. There is no evidence of a link to allergy and these patients are not prone to skin infections.

Psoriasis

All cases of psoriasis classically present as erythematous papules and plaques with silver scales. There are five different subtypes of psoriasis:

1. chronic plaque psoriasis – occurs in 80% of cases
2. guttate psoriasis
3. pustular psoriasis
4. erythrodermic psoriasis
5. palmar plantar pustulosis

Psoriasis is an immune-mediated process with a strong genetic basis in which certain cytokines (e.g. interferon-α, interleukins IL-12 and IL-23) induce inflammation and recruit T cells to the skin. These T cells lead to hyperproliferation of keratinocytes and the thickened plaques of psoriasis.

Psoriasis may be exacerbated or triggered by environmental factors such as sunlight or infection – streptococcal or HIV. Psychological stress, smoking and some drugs, including lithium, antimalarials and angiotensin-converting enzyme inhibitors, may also exacerbate disease.

Psoriasis is associated with a seronegative arthritis in up to 40% of patients and with inflammatory bowel disease. Patients with psoriasis also have an increased risk of cardiovascular disease.

Clinical insight

All patients with psoriasis should be assessed for signs of arthritis and cardiovascular disease.

Chronic plaque psoriasis

The prevalence of psoriasis is estimated at 2.2%, it can occur at any age but most cases present before the age of 35 years.

Important differential diagnoses to exclude are:

- **mycosis fungoides:** often misdiagnosed as psoriasis for many years; consider if treatment is refractory and in non-typical presentations
- **Bowen's disease:** consider in patients with actinic damage and solitary plaques
- **tinea corporis:** usually starts as an isolated area and as a patch rather than a plaque

Clinical features

Clinical features of chronic plaque psoriasis include:

- well-demarcated erythematous plaques with silver scales distributed symmetrically over the body (**Figure 9.6**); gentle scraping accentuates the scale and vigorous scraping causes pinpoint bleeding (Auspitz's sign)

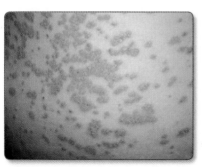

Figure 9.6 Psoriasis.

- fissuring within plaques on the joint lines
- extensor site involvement – elbows, knees, back, buttocks
- ear and periumbilical involvement
- classic nail changes – onycholysis, pitting, brown discoloration

There may also be plaques in the scalp with marked scaling.

The disease extent and severity are measured using the psoriasis area and severity index. This rates disease according to erythema, plaque thickness and scaling.

Diagnosis is usually made on the basis of the the clinical findings; rarely a biopsy is required. If this is the case see Chapter 18.

Treatment

A full explanation about the chronic nature of the disease should be given to the patient and reassurance that this is not an infectious process. Consider a patient's cardiovascular risk when the psoriasis is severe. Ask about joint pain or swelling and refer appropriately. Ask directly about any social and psychological effects of the psoriasis.

Treatment for mild-to-moderate disease is with regular emollients to control scaling. Short-term topical therapy with moderate-potency **topical steroids** and **topical vitamin D** analogue preparations should be used daily to control flares. Aggressive use of topical steroids can lead to a flare of pustular psoriasis.

Phototherapy This is a second-line treatment for extensive, widespread disease. Narrow-band UVB phototherapy should be offered to patients with disease uncontrolled by topical therapies. Photochemotherapy with a photosensitising agent (psoralen) can be used in combination with UVA in resistant disease; long-term complications include an increased risk of skin cancer.

Treatment for moderate disease is as above but with the addition of systemic immunosuppression using agents such as **ciclosporin, methotrexate** and **acitretin**, usually started by a dermatologist.

Severe disease refractory to systemic therapy may be treated with **systemic biologic therapies** which use molecules that block specific steps in the development of psoriasis, such as anti-tumour necrosis factor (TNF) agents (inflximab, etanercept, adalimumab) or IL-12/IL-23 antagonists (ustekinumab). Biologic drugs require close patient monitoring. Currently, these agents are all administered by injection or infusion.

Psoriasis area and severity index scores should be taken pre-treatment and at intervals during treatment to ascertain efficacy.

Guttate psoriasis

This is a distinctive acute eruption; it is more common in individuals aged <35 years and is often associated with a streptococcal throat infection. There is a genetic predisposition to the disease and there may be a positive family history for psoriasis.

Clinical features

In most cases there is a 2- to 3-week antecedent history of a streptococcal pharyngitis. The anti-streptolysin O titre should be assessed in all suspected cases.

There is an acute onset of multiple, small, drop-like, pink plaques and papules on the trunk and proximal extremities, which may spread to the face. There may be a fine scale present on older lesions. There are usually no nail changes.

Important differentials are **pityriasis rosea, tinea corporis** and **secondary syphilis**.

Treatment

The rash usually resolves within a few months and emollients are used by all patients. Some patients may go on to develop chronic plaque psoriasis; this tends to be those with a family history. If treatment is required a short course of narrow-band UVB phototherapy is the optimum treatment for guttate psoriasis.

Generalised pustular psoriasis

This is a rare, severe eruptive form of psoriasis accompanied by fever; it can be life threatening. Recognised triggers of the disease are infection, use of potent topical steroid, withdrawal of oral corticosteroids, drugs (e.g. antibiotics, salicylates) and pregnancy. In many cases no cause is identified. The differential diagnosis includes AGEP (see page 120).

Clinical features

The following clinical features may be present:

- Patients are unwell with malaise and fever; in some cases they have diarrhoea.
- There may be a widespread acute erythema with rapid spread of multiple pustules (sterile) (**Figure 9.7**).
- Liver function may be deranged and patient may be anaemic.

Treatment

Patients should be urgently admitted to hospital. They require intensive supportive therapy for fluid and temperature regulation. Regular emollients and bland compresses can soothe the skin.

Systemic steroids are not used; agents including ciclosporin, methotrexate and acitretin have all been used to good effect. There is increasing use of biologic agents, such as adalimumab and infliximab, to treat this condition.

Clinical insight

Avoid potent topical steroids in patients with psoriasis because their withdrawal may lead to generalised pustular psoriasis.

Erythrodermic psoriasis
See page 265.

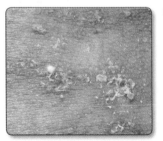

Figure 9.7 Pustular psoriasis.

Palmar plantar pustulosis

This type of psoriasis predominantly affects the palms and soles; it is a chronic condition that is strongly associated with smoking and more common in women.

Clinical features

There is a symmetrical eruption of yellow–brown pustules and vesicles localised to the palms and soles with background erythema. The vesicle and pustules become dry and scaly. Approximately 15% of patients have plaques of psoriasis elsewhere.

Treatment

Mild disease can be treated with topical agents. Thick emollients should be applied frequently. Coal tar may be applied at night under cotton gloves which can improve the scale and inflammation. Ultrapotent topical steroid ointment may be applied for 2–4 weeks to the palms and soles to reduce itching and inflammation.

Severe disease usually requires phototherapy with topical psoralen and ultraviolet (UV) A, or systemic agents such as acitretin, methotrexate or isotretinoin. Biologic agents such as infliximab and adalimumab may also be used.

9.4 Clinical scenario

A 70-year-old man presents with a 5-day history of blisters and malaise. His skin has been itchy for about 2–3 months before the onset of the blisters. There is no history of previous skin disease. The patient has hypertension and had a previous cerebrovascular accident; he has been on a calcium channel blocker for many years. He has not taken any over-the-counter medications.

On examination there are multiple, intact, tense blisters on an inflamed base on his trunk, arms and thighs. They measured between 1 and 4 cm and have associated excoriation. There is no involvement of the eyes, mouth or genitals. His nails are normal.

Diagnostic approach

Differential diagnoses for an inflammatory blistering disorder include:

- **drug-induced blistering:** no clear history of a drug trigger
- **Stevens–Johnson syndrome/toxic epidermal necrolysis (TEN):** absence of mucosal involvement excludes Stevens–Johnson syndrome. Blisters intact; no TEN at present
- **bullous lupus erythematosus:** no prior history of lupus erythematosus (LE), and no clinical evidence of LE elsewhere, so this is less likely to be the diagnosis
- **autoimmune blistering disorders** (e.g. pemphigus vulgaris, bullous pemphigoid): no mucosal involvement so makes pemphigus vulgaris less likely

The patient's age and clinical presentation make bullous pemphigoid the most likely diagnosis. See below for investigations and management.

9.5 Bullous diseases

Bullous pemphigoid

This is an autoimmune blistering disease, which most commonly occurs in patients aged >60 years (mean age 80 years). Autoantibodies bind to antigens at the dermoepidermal junction, leading to subepidermal blister formation. The autoantigen is a type XVII collagen. Differential diagnoses include dermatitis herpetiformis, bullous LE and pemphigus vulgaris.

Clinical features

Before the development of blisters patients may have an intensely pruritic eruption with a rash. The prodromal rash may be papular, urticarial or eczematous; patients go on to develop widespread, tense blisters on an erythematous or urticarial base (**Figure 9.8**). There is sparing of the mucous membranes. The bullae heal without scarring.

Skin biopsy from an area of blistering is required to make the diagnosis. Lesional skin should be sent for haematoxylin and eosin (H&E) staining in formalin. Perilesional tissues should be sent for immunofluorescence (IMF) studies in Michel's medium, which enable detection of autoantibodies at the dermoepider-

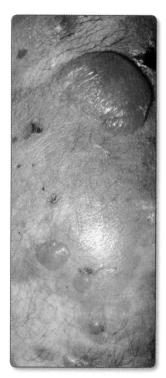

Figure 9.8 Bullous pemphigoid.

mal junction. Bloods should be performed to establish baseline full blood count (FBC), renal and liver function, along with an autoimmune screen to exclude lupus.

Treatment

The following are the initial general measures:

- Blisters should be ruptured using a sterile needle but the roof of the blister should be left in place.
- A potent topical steroid (clobetasol) can be applied to lesions and any inflamed skin if there is localised disease.

The main aim of treatment is to reduce blister formation. Disease is often chronic and a systemic agent may be required to control blister formation. Patients on systemic treatment require close

Clinical insight

Bullous pemphigoid presents with intact blisters, and pemphigus vulgaris with erosions at the site of ruptured blisters.

monitoring. Use of aggressive treatment regimens may put the patient's life more at risk than the underlying disease. Systemic Immunosuppression is initially with oral prednisolone (0.75–1.0 mg/kg per day); calcium and vitamin D supplements should be given as well. This regimen is effective in 60–90% of patients within 1 month. Although there is little evidence for their use, azathioprine, mycophenolate mofetil and methotrexate are commonly used as steroid-sparing agents.

Pemphigus

This describes a group of autoimmune disorders in which there is superficial blistering of the mucosa and skin. Circulating IgG autoantibodies bind to keratinocytes in the epidermis, leading to intraepidermal blister formation. The group comprises:
- pemphigus vulgaris, the most common variant
- pemphigus foliaceus, skin-only lesions in association with desmoglein 1
- paraneoplastic pemphigus in association with a tumour (see page 203)

Clinical features

Pemphigus vulgaris can occur at any age but is more common in patients aged >30 years. The disease appears to be triggered by environmental factors such as drugs (captopril, penicillamine), immunisations or stress.

Skin lesions are flaccid blisters that rupture easily; in fact they rupture so easily that usually only inflammatory, painful erosions are visible on the skin (**Figure 9.9**). Blisters are Nikolsky positive – mechanical pressure at the edge of a blister induces further blister formation. There is mucosal involvement (**Figure 9.10**). Patients report pain on swallowing; again usually only erosions are present. Blisters can occur on the conjunctiva, upper gastrointestinal tract and genitalia.

Pemphigus foliaceus presents in the same way but with only skin lesions.

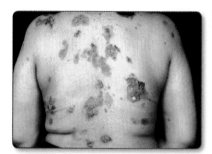

Figure 9.9 Pemphigus vulgaris on the chest.

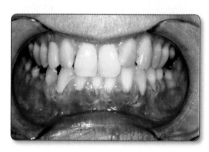

Figure 9.10 Pemphigus vulgaris in the mouth.

Investigations

General investigations such as FBC, urea and electrolytes, liver function tests, chest radiograph and urinalysis are warranted. A skin biopsy should be taken from the edge of a blister. Direct and indirect IMF should be performed. Enzyme-linked immunoassays (ELISAs) can be performed on the serum to identify desmoglein 1 and desmoglein 3 (autoantibodies involved).

Management

General measures should be advised, including emollients to protect the skin barrier, oral care with a soft diet and soft toothbrush, and ophthalmology involvement. Mild oral disease can be managed by direct application of beclometasone using an asthma inhaler

Systemic corticosteroids, up to a dose of 1 mg/kg per day, usually results in remission in 6 weeks. Steroid-sparing agents for long-term control are usually azathioprine, mycophenolate mofetil and dapsone. For severe disease refractory to other treatments, rituximab and plasma exchange have been used.

Dermatitis herpetiformis

This autoimmune blistering disease is associated with coeliac disease. Evidence suggests these conditions have a shared pathogenesis involving gluten sensitivity. In both the immune response to components of gluten leads to inflammation. Dermatitis herpetiformis occurs most commonly in northern European patients and is seen more frequently in men than in women, with an age of onset around 40 years. Differential diagnoses include atopic dermatitis, scabies and insect bites.

Clinical features

Dermatitis herpetiformis is an intensely itchy, bullous eruption usually affecting the extensor surfaces. Lesions are grouped papules and vesicles which rarely resolve spontaneously. Patients may have a history of autoimmune thyroid disease, vitiligo and type 1 diabetes, and usually a history of associated coeliac disease.

Investigations

The following investigations should be undertaken to confirm the diagnosis:
- skin biopsy for H&E which shows subepidermal blistering and direct IMF which shows IgA deposition in the dermal papillae
- serology for coeliac disease (positive in 90% of patients)
- blood tests to look for anaemia; test for iron deficiency

Clinical insight

Nearly *all* patients with dermatitis herpetiformis will have coeliac disease, so it is important that this is diagnosed to avoid complications related to coeliac disease such as gluten ataxia and non-Hodgkin's lymphoma

Treatment

A strict gluten-free diet is started; this allows easier control of the skin symptoms and reduces the medications required to treat the skin. Drug treatment is with dapsone, which can lead to a rapid resolution of dermatitis herpetiformis within a few days. Once there good dietary control has been obtained, the dapsone may be stopped.

9.6 Clinical scenario

A 59-year-old woman presents with a 4-year history of persistent facial redness on his nose and cheeks. She also reports red 'spots' that come and go with the redness. The facial rash is more noticeable after exercise, in warm environments or when she has had alcohol. The rash has never been itchy and is not worse in summertime or on sunny holidays. The patient had eczema as a child and reports having dandruff intermittently. She was recently diagnosed with hypertension, for which she takes bendroflumethazide. She is otherwise well but feels embarrassed by the persistent rash on her face.

Examination

On examination there is patchy erythema in a 'butterfly' distribution on her nose and cheeks, with a number of telangiectasias (**Figure 9.11**). There are no comedones, papules, pustules or vesicles, and the rash is not scaly. There is no evidence of excoriation.

Diagnostic approach – 'the red face' (Figure 9.12)

The differential for the red face includes:
- allergic contact dermatitis
- atopic dermatitis

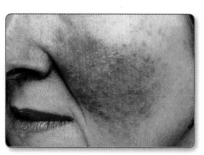

Figure 9.11 Rosacea.

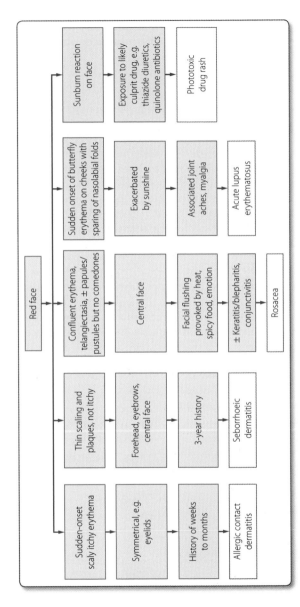

Figure 9.12 Diagnostic flowchart – the red face.

- rosacea
- seborrhoeic dermatitis
- systemic lupus erythematosus (SLE)
  Clues from the history and examination are:
- the rash is not itchy: makes allergic contact dermatitis or atopic dermatitis unlikely
- the rash is not scaly and does not involve forehead or melo-labial folds: makes seborrhoeic dermatitis unlikely
- 'butterfly' rash: this phrase is commonly associated with the facial rash of SLE. However, the rash in this case is not photosensitive (no seasonal variation) and there are no systemic features of SLE
- exacerbating factors (exercise and alcohol): suggest rosacea
- facial erythema and telangiectasia: suggest rosacea

The most likely diagnosis, based on the history and clinical features, is erythematotelangiectatic rosacea.

> **Clinical insight**
>
> The cause of a 'red face' may be found with patch testing, mycology studies, lupus serology and/or phototesting.

9.7 Adnexal skin disease

These diseases involve the hair follicle and sweat gland unit.

Acne vulgaris

This disorder of the pilosebaceous unit occurs in almost all adolescents. Androgen hormones stimulate sebum production and are a factor in the development of acne. Predisposition to acne is inherited from family members. Stress is thought to exacerbate it but the role of diet is unclear. New-onset acne in adults may be due to androgen-secreting tumours.

Differential diagnoses include rosacea, drug-induced acne, perioral dermatitis and sebaceous hyperplasia.

Acne can have a profound effect on self-esteem and it is important to treat it quickly and efficiently.

> **Clinical insight**
>
> *Propionibacterium acnes* proliferation has a role in the development of acne.

Clinical features

Acne predominantly affects the face, and in some cases the back and chest. The skin is usually greasy; the severity of presentation varies widely.

Patients may have just some of the following features:
- non-inflammatory lesions:
  - closed comedones – white heads
  - open comedones – blackheads
- inflammatory lesions: erythematous papules, pustules and nodules
- scarring: pits or atrophic dips in the skin; in patients with a tendency to keloid, scarring can become keloidal

Acne fulminans is a serious variant of acne requiring urgent attention. Patients present with large inflamed nodules and crusting, associated fevers and arthralgias.

> ### Clinical insight
> Acne fulminans is a systemic disorder requiring treatment with systemic steroids 0.5–1mg/kg per day.

Treatment

Treatment aims are to decrease follicular proliferation, sebum production, *Propionibacterium acnes* proliferation and inflammation.

The treatment required depends on the type of acne and type of skin that the patient has; the treatment may be topical or systemic depending on the severity of the acne. Antiacne medications have different mechanisms of action.

Topical preparations Comedonal lesions: both retinoids and salicylic acid 10% are effective. Benzoyl peroxide also reduces sebum production and decreases colonisation of skin by *P. acnes*.

Inflammatory lesions: topical antibiotics with clindamycin or erythromycin can be effective.

Systemic treatment This may be used in combination with topical preparations. Systemic treatment is initiated earlier in patients presenting with scarring:
- Antibiotic therapy: doxycycline and lymecycline are usually considered first line

- Anti-androgen therapy: in women this is predominantly an oestrogenic oral contraceptive
- Oral isotretinoin: this is highly effective but requires specialist initiation; it is teratogenic

Rosacea

This facial dermatosis is common in patients with type I/II skin. Usually it occurs in patients in middle age. Genetics, UV exposure, hypersensitivity of cutaneous vasculature and innate immune response to microorganisms are all thought to contribute to this disease.

Differential diagnoses include seborrhoeic dermatitis, acute lupus erythematosus and acne vulgaris.

Clinical features

The main variants of rosacea recognised are:
- **erythematotelangiectatic:** persistent erythema of the central face, prominent telangiectasias and flushing
- **papulopustular:** persistent erythema of the central face, papules and pustules
- **phymatous:** thickened skin with prominent pores, classically affecting the nose, termed 'rhinophyma'
- **ocular:** dry, gritty eyes with burning and stinging secondary to conjunctivitis, blepharitis and keratitis

Hot drinks, spicy foods, alcohol, sun exposure, stress and anxiety are frequently reported as disease exacerbators.

Treatment

The following are treatment for the different variants:
- **Facial erythema:** patients should avoid recognised triggers and use high sun protection factor sunscreen.
- **Papulopustular disease:** use topical antimicrobials (metronidazole) and topical retinoids (azelaic acid). A 12-week trial of oral tetracyclines can be used, or low-dose oral isotretinoin for disease refractory to antibiotics.
- **Phymatous rosacea:** low-dose Isotretinoin and laser ablation may be helpful.

Hidradenitis suppurativa

This is a chronic inflammatory skin disease involving the hair follicles. It is also known as acne inversa. It affects between 1 and 4% of the population and is more common in those of African–Caribbean descent. There is a genetic susceptibility; androgens, smoking, obesity, mechanical stress and bacteria are all thought to play a role in causing disease.

Clinical features

The axilla, groins, perineum and inframammary zones are affected.

- **Inflammatory nodules:** these last for weeks to months and are intermittently extremely painful and drain pustular discharge. They are driven by an inflammatory response rather than infection. Usually they are multiple and affect the sites outlined above.
- **Sinus tracts:** these are formed when nodules join together. They are below the skin and filled with serosanguineous fluid or pus. They may not always be palpable (**Figure 9.13**).
- **Scarring:** hypertrophic scars occur with chronic inflammation.
- In severe, poorly controlled disease, **fistulae** into the bladder, rectum and urethra may occur.
- Patients are at risk of developing **cutaneous squamous cell carcinoma** at sites of chronically active inflammation.
- **Disease severity** is variable and graded according to Hurley's system (**Table 9.2**).

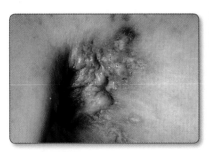

Figure 9.13 Hurley's stage III hidradenitis suppurativa.

Stage	Characteristics
Stage I	Abscess formation without sinus tracts or scarring
Stage II	Recurrent abscesses with sinus tracts and scarring
Stage III	Diffuse involvement with abscesses, interconnecting tracts and scarring

Table 9.2 Hurley's stages of hidradenitis suppurativa

Discharge is often malodorous and inflammation around the groins and perineal area can make it difficult to sit down or walk. Patients are often extremely embarrassed and find it difficult to work and have relationships. They may become **depressed** quite easily and should be treated for this accordingly.

Investigations

The diagnosis is a clinical one and skin biopsy is not normally required to make a diagnosis of hidradenitis suppurativa.

Bacterial swabs may be useful to establish colonising microorganisms. These may contribute to chronic inflammation and should be treated in active disease. Magnetic resonance imaging is useful to assess the extent of sinus tract disease.

Bloods show anaemia of chronic disease and markedly elevated inflammatory markers.

Treatment

Weight loss and smoking cessation should be recommended to the patient. Other treatments include chlorhexidine wash, intra-lesional triamcinolone and surgical excision of affected areas.

Depending on the severity of disease systemic treatments are usually tried in the following order.

- **Oral antibiotics:** lymecycline, clindamycin and rifampicin often used
- **Antiandrogen therapy:** estradiol and cyproterone acetate, finasteride
- **Retinoids:** isotretinoin and acitretin

> **Clinical insight**
>
> Hidradenitis suppurativa is not primarily an infectious process and requires antiinflammatory treatment.

- **Corticosteroids:** prednisolone, which may be useful in resolving severe exacerbations
- **Immunosuppression:** ciclosporin, mycophenolate mofetil, azathioprine
- **Anti-TNFα inhibitors:** e.g. infliximab, adalimumab

Infectious diseases

Cutaneous infection is a common cause for referral to a dermatologist. The pathogen may be bacterial, viral or fungal. Clinicians should be alert to conditions predisposing to cutaneous infection, e.g. eczema, diabetes, malignancy and underlying immunosuppression.

10.1 Clinical scenario

A 72-year-old man presents with a 2-day history of a painful, blistering rash on his abdomen; this was preceded by a burning sensation before onset of the rash. He has no fever but feels exhausted.

Diagnostic approach

The acute nature of a rash that is confined to one location on the body may suggest an infective cause or a contact dermatitis. Continue to a full history relating to allergy and a full skin examination.

Examination and investigations

On examination there are grouped vesicles on a swollen erythematous base visible on the left T10 dermatome on the anterior abdomen only.

Diagnostic approach

Varicella-zoster virus reactivation (herpes zoster) is the most common cause of a painful, acute, vesicular eruption in a dermatomal distribution. Confirmation is with a viral swab of the lesions, although such swabs are often negative because the viruses are difficult to detect from the scrapes. A polymerase chain reaction assay is more sensitive.

Treatment is with aciclovir 800 mg fives times a day for 7 days, started within 72 hours of rash onset.

10.2 Bacterial infections

Impetigo

This is a very common superficial bacterial infection of the skin; it usually occurs in children. It is more common in hot climates due to sweating and insect bites damaging the skin barrier. Patients with eczema are also at high risk of developing it.

Clinical features

Impetigo may be bullous or non-bullous (more common). Non-bullous lesions start as small papules on an inflammatory base which evolve into golden crusts over the course of 7 days (**Figure 10.1**). Bullous lesions are thin-roofed blisters over an erythematous crusted base which tend to rupture spontaneously. Impetigo usually affects the trunk.

Investigations

Skin swabs should be taken from the affected sites. Infection is usually caused by *Staphylococcus aureus* or group A streptococcus.

Treatment

- All patients should have local treatment to cleanse the skin at the affected site.
- Towels should not be shared with family members due to the highly contagious nature of impetigo.
- Topical therapy is the treatment of choice (e.g. fusidic acid, mupirocin).

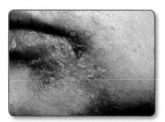

Figure 10.1 Impetigo.

- Oral antibiotics should be used for bullous lesions or if a large area is involved.
- If *Streptococcus* spp. is cultured, patients should be followed up within 3–4 weeks and have a urine dipstick test performed because they are at risk of developing poststreptococccal glomerulonephritis.

Folliculitis

This is due to obstruction of the pilosebaceous glands and may or may not include infection. *Staphylococcus aureus* is the most common infection; *Pseudomonas* spp. can occur associated with use of hot tubs. Fungal folliculitis due to *Candida* and *Trichophyton* spp. can also occur, particularly in the beard area.

Clinical features

Clinical features include multiple pruritic erythematous papules and pustules. These commonly occur at the site of repeated shaving or epilation.

Investigations

Bacterial swabs should be taken from the skin and nose to establish the colonising organism. *S. aureus* is the most common.

Treatment

Folliculitis usually resolves spontaneously. The following general measures should be observed in all patients:

- reduce frequency of shaving and shave in the direction of hair follicle growth
- maintain good skin hygiene and use separate towels from other family members
- if necessary topical therapy can be given (fusidic acid, mupirocin)
- treat nasal carriage

Abscesses and furuncles

These are deep-seated infections within the base of the hair follicle. Scarring is more common in this type of folliculitis.

Clinical features

The features include:
- tender, fluctuant painful nodules that may be white/yellow in colour
- inflamed erythematous base
- fever and malaise, which may indicate systemic involvement
- lesions commonly occurring on the neck, face, axillae and buttocks

Investigation

Bacterial swabs from a pustule and the nose should be taken.

Treatment

> **Clinical insight**
>
> Cutaneous infection on periorbital and nasal skin carries a risk of septic embolism and cavernous sinus thrombosis.

Incision and drainage (I&D) under local anaesthetic help to relieve pain and aid recovery. A 7-day course of broad-spectrum antibiotics (e.g. co-amoxiclav) is given after I&D. In severe or recurrent cases antibiotic therapy may be required for 6 weeks.

Cellulitis and erysipelas

Cellulitis occurs mainly in middle-aged individuals and erysipelas in children and elderly people. The risk factors are given

Risk factor	Example
Impaired skin barrier	Insect bites, intravenous drug use, eczema, trauma
Infection	Tinea pedis, varicella-zoster
Venous insufficiency	Oedema, previous DVT or vein stripping
Lymphatic insufficiency	Post-surgery or DVT
Comorbidities	Diabetes, lymphoedema, malignancy, immunodeficiency
DVT, deep vein thrombosis.	

Table 10.1 Risk factors for cellulitis and erysipelas

in **Table 10.1**. Erysipelas is usually caused by β-haemolytic *Streptoccocus* and cellulitis by either β-haemolytic *Streptoccocus* or *Staphlococcus aureus*.

Differential diagnoses include contact dermatitis, deep vein thrombosis (DVT), drug reactions and insect bites.

Clinical features

The clinical features of **erysipelas** include:
- infection in **superficial dermis** and lymphatics
- abrupt onset over about 24 hours with malaise, fever and chills
- localised painful erythema with **sharp demarcation** between affected and unaffected skin (**Figure 10.2**)
- legs and face as common site of involvement
- infection, usually unilateral

The clinical features of **cellulitis** include:
- deeper infection involving the deep dermis and subcutaneous fat
- onset slower than erysipelas and takes days to evolve
- patients present with diffuse painful erythema and swelling; may be associated pustules, vesicles or bullae

> **Clinical insight**
>
> Both cellulitis and erysipelas are predominantly **unilateral** diseases.

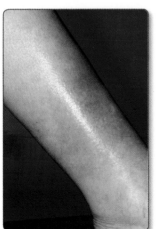

Figure 10.2 Erysipelas.

- legs the most common site of involvement
- infection usually unilateral

Investigations

Investigations should include:
- bloods: elevated white cell count and inflammatory markers
- bacterial swabs taken from affected areas
- mycology skin scrapings or toenail clippings
- blood cultures if there is evidence of systemic infection

Treatment

Acute infection Empirical intravenous antibiotic therapy is given. Regimens include flucloxacillin and benzylpenicillin or vancomycin or cefotaxime. If there is an improvement after 48 hours patients may be switched to a 7- to 14-day course of oral therapy.

Recurrent infection Patients are treated as above and risk factors such as venous eczema, tinea pedis and lymphoedema are identified and treated.

Prophylaxis Long-term antibiotic therapy (12 months) with low-dose phenoxymethylpenicillin (e.g. 250 mg twice daily) is helpful in reducing recurrence.

Erythrasma

This is a chronic superficial infection of the intertriginous skin caused by *Corynebacterium minutissimum*. It may be a presenting sign of diabetes and is more common in obese, elderly and immunocompromised individuals. Differential diagnoses include seborrhoeic dermatitis, dermatophyte infection and 'inverse' psoriasis.

Clinical features

The clinical features include:
- scaly erythematous brown plaques with macerated skin change (**Figure 10.3**)
- skin between the toes and in axillae, and groin involved

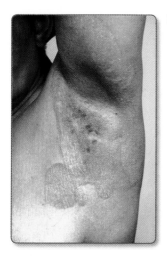
Figure 10.3 Erythrasma.

Investigations

Investigations for erythrasma should include:

- Wood's lamp (365 nm) examination of affected areas, which shows coral-red fluorescence
- mycology skin scrapings to exclude dermatophye infection
- bacterial swabs

Treatment

Localised disease Topical therapy is with antiseptic or topical antibiotic agents such as fusidic acid and benzoylperoxide.

Widespread disease Give oral treatment with a macrolide antibiotic or a tetracycline if there is a history of allergy to macrolides.

Meningococcal infection

Neisseria meningitidis is the leading cause of bacterial meningitis in children. Systemic infection has a mortality rate of 10–15% despite antibiotic treatment.

Meningococcal sepsis is associated with particular skin features which should alert the clinician to the severity of the infection.

Clinical features

Clinical features of meningococcal sepsis include the following.

- There may be a transient rash resembling a viral exanthem early in disease
- Pallor or mottling of the skin is an early sign of systemic infection; leg pain and cold hands/feet are also early signs of systemic infection
- There is a petechial rash of non-blanching violaceous macules (**Figure 10.4**)
- Purpura fulminans (see page 271) is a serious complication of meningococcal disease
- Patients are extremely unwell with hypotension, tachycardia and fever, and often multiorgan failure

Investigations and treatment

In suspected cases of meningoccal infection:

- obtain blood cultures promptly
- give empirical intravenous antibiotics immediately after cultures have been taken; third-generation cephalosporins are usually used
- do not delay administration of antibiotics for any other investigation, e.g. lumbar puncture
- organ support may be required, e.g. inotropes and haemo-filtration

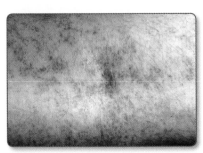

Figure 10.4 Petechial rash.

- cover breaches in the skin barrier carefully with thick barrier agents to prevent secondary infection

Lyme disease

This is a tick-borne disease caused by borrelia spirochetes, most commonly *Borrelia burgdorferi*. The ticks live on hosts such as deer, and humans may contract the disease when they are bitten by ticks of *Ixodes* sp. Usually patients have visited a high-risk area, although they may not recall having been bitten.

Clinical features

The clinical features depend on the stage of disease at which the patient presents. These stages of Lyme disease are summarised in **Table 10.2**.

Stage	Clinical feature	Symptoms
Early localised	Erythema migrans (**Figure 10.5**)	Appears at site 7–14 days after tick bite Annular erythema expands with central clearing Associated with fatigue, headache, anorexia, myalgia, arthralgia or fever
Early disseminated	Borrelial lymphocytoma	Solitary, bluish-red swelling Found on nipples in adults or ears in children Manifests neurologically as cranial nerve palsies, peripheral neuropathy or meningitis Patients may have atrioventricular node block and pericarditis
Late	Acrodermatitis chronica atrophicans	Occurs years after initial infection Bluish-red skin change with swelling Edge of the lesion will advance and the erythema resolves Lesion becomes atrophic and subcutaneous veins are visible May have oligoarthritis in large joints, polyneuropathy and/or encephalitis

Table 10.2 Stages of Lyme disease and their symptoms

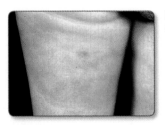

Figure 10.5 Erythema chronica migrans.

Investigations

A two-step method is required to look for antibodies to *Borrelia* sp. The initial enzyme immunoassay has a high false-positive rate; the second step test uses immunoblotting. It is important to record the date of exposure or tick bite on requests for serology, as antibodies may not be present in the first 4–6 weeks of infection.

Treatment

A 3-week course of oral doxycycline is the treatment of choice. Amoxicillin and cefuroxime are options if the patient has a tetracycline allergy. Intravenous treatment may be required if disease is severe or refractory to oral treatment.

Syphilis

This is a sexually transmitted infection caused by the spirochaete *Treponema pallidum*. The disease is divided into three stages: primary, secondary and tertiary syphilis.

> **Clinical insight**
>
> Patients must be tested for HIV if syphilis is suspected.

Clinical features

The clinical features of primary, secondary and tertiary syphilis are shown in **Table 10.3**. Patients with tertiary syphilis are also at risk of developing:

- aortic valve regurgitation, left cardiac failure and syphilitic aneurysms of the ascending thoracic aorta
- paresis and tabes dorsalis

Stage	Clinical features
Primary	Occurs 3 weeks after infection Solitary papule develops on genitals; this ulcerates (chancre) and is associated with regional lymphadenopathy Chancres are painless and resolve within 6 weeks
Secondary	Occurs within a few months of infection Widespread papulosquamous rash affecting palms and soles (**Figure 10.6**) May be a non-scarring, 'moth-eaten' alopecia affecting the scalp, eyebrows and beard area Grey/white plaques (condylomata lata) may develop close to the site of primary infection
Tertiary	Occurs months or years after initial infection, during which time syphilis has been latent Gummatous syphilis: granulomatous nodular lesions that ulcerate (**Figure 10.7**); gummas may also be present in visceral organs and bones

Table 10.3 Stages of syphilis

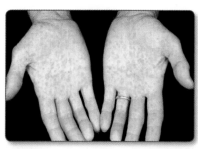

Figure 10.6 Secondary syphilis.

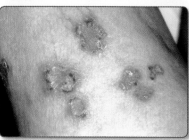

Figure 10.7 Gummatous syphilis.

Investigations

Treponema pallidum cannot be cultured and the diagnosis has to be made on the basis of serology:

- Non-treponemal tests: Venereal Disease Research Laboratory is the best known of these and is used as an initial screening test.
- Treponemal tests: these are used as confirmatory tests and examples include the fluorescent treponemal antibody–absorbed (FTA-Abs).

Treatment

Penicillin is the treatment of choice. Macrolides, tetracyclines and cephalosporins may be used in penicillin-allergic patients.

10.3 Viral infections

Viral infections are a common cause of mucosal and skin infections; they may present in the skin alone or be associated with systemic disease.

See Chapter 14 for information on warts, molluscum, varicella-zoster virus, measles and parvovirus.

Herpes zoster – shingles

Varicella-zoster virus (VZV) causes chickenpox as a primary infection before establishing lifelong latent infection. Reactivation results in herpes zoster (shingles).

Clinical features

The clinical features include:

- sudden onset of vesicular erythematous eruption
- pustules, crusting and pain
- involvement of a single dermatome in immunocompetent hosts (**Figure 10.8**); multiple dermatomes may be involved in immunosuppressed individuals
- post-herpetic neuralgia following resolution of the rash

Clinical insight

Herpes zoster involving the trigeminal ophthalmic dermatome or nasal tip may lead to sight-threatening herpes keratitis. Urgent ophthalmology review is required.

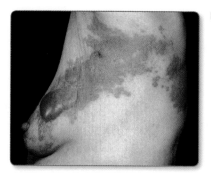

Figure 10.8 Shingles.

Investigations

These include viral swab for culture and polymerase chain reaction (PCR) testing to identify VZV.

Treatment

The treatment options include:
- aciclovir, valaciclovir or famciclovir
- analgesia, which should be given for acute neuritis
- corticosteroids, which are advocated by some to help prevent development of postherpetic neuralgia

HSV-1

The herpes simplex virus type 1 (HSV-1, also known as herpes labialis) mainly affects the skin and oral mucosa. The virus lies latent after primary infection and can be reactivated, leading to recurrent infection, most commonly 'cold sores'.

Clinical features

Clinical features include:
- primary infection:
  - oral: adults or children may develop fever, pharyngitis and painful vesicles on the lips and oral mucosa; infections last for between 5 and 7 days

> ### Clinical insight
>
> HSV-1 oral infection in a patient with facial eczema can lead to eczema herpeticum.

  – cutaneous: multiple grouped vesicles on an inflammatory base; lesions last for up to 14 days and patients are infectious during this period
- recurrent Infection:
  – oral: painful vesicular erythematous lesions at the angles of the mouth; they may be preceded by a tingling sensation; these are 'cold' sores, which typically crust over and last for a week
  – cutaneous: grouped vesicles usually occur at site of primary infection; they may be induced by sunlight, stress or immunosuppression

Clinical insight

Erythema multiforme (EM) is an immune-mediated response, usually to an infection. Common causes are commonly herpes simplex or *Mycoplasma pneumonia*. It is characterised by target like skin lesions. These have a dusky erythematous centre surrounded by a pale ring of oedema and pink border (**Figure 10.9**). EM affects the palms, soles and often the oral and genital mucosa.

HSV-2

This virus usually leads to disease of the genital mucosa and is transmitted sexually. It mainly affects the genital mucosa.

Clinical features

These include the following:

- Primary infection: patients may be asymptomatic or have painful genital ulcers with associated fever, dysuria and lymphadenopathy; signs and symptoms may persist for 3 weeks
- Recurrent infection: vesicular or ulcerative genital lesions occur and last for around 10 days; during this time patients are infectious

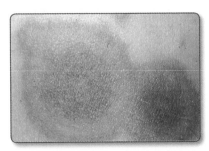

Figure 10.9 Erythema multiforme.

Investigations
Viral swabs for PCR studies can isolate the subtype of HSV.

Treatment
Oral aciclovir, valaciclovir or famciclovir for 7–10 days may be used in immunocompetent patients.

Patients with recurrent disease or HSV-induced erythema multiforme may require continuous therapy for 6 months to 1 year. Immunosuppressed patients are at risk of developing systemic disease, with possible complications including encephalitis. Intravenous treatment may be required.

Human immunodeficiency virus
A seroconversion rash occurs in up to 80% of patients with HIV. Patients feel unwell with fever, myalgia, lymphadenopathy and a morbilliform exanthem. The rash occurs about 4 weeks after the virus was contracted.

Many cutaneous diseases are associated with established HIV infection, including seborrhoeic dermatitis, oropharyngeal candidiasis, herpes zoster, herpes simplex, psoriasis, molluscum contagiosum, cutaneous tuberculosis (TB), eosinophilic folliculitis and psoriasis, and Kaposi's sarcoma.

> **Clinical insight**
>
> Kaposi's sarcoma is a tumour caused by human herpesvirus 8; the tumours are purple brown in colour and can occur in immunodeficiency. Always request HIV testing and arrange a dermatology review.

10.4 Fungal infections
Fungi can be divided into dermatophytes, yeasts and moulds, all of which cause cutaneous infection.

Dermatophytes
The most common cutaneous fungal infection is caused by dermatophytes: *Trichophyton*, *Epidermophyton* and *Microsporum* spp. These organisms survive on keratin, found in abundance in the hair, nails and skin.

Clinical features

These include the following.

- **Tinea pedis (athlete's foot):** itchy erythematous scaly erosions occur with macerated skin in the toe web spaces.
- **Tinea corporis:** lesions are erythematous, scaly, circular or oval patches or plaques (**Figure 10.10**). These expand outwards with central clearing and an 'advancing' scaly edge. Parents of children with tinea capitis are at risk, as are athletes who have close skin-to-skin contact.
- **Tinea capitis:** occurs in children most commonly. The scalp is initially scaly with a well-demarcated patch of erythema. The patch expands over the course of a few weeks and hairs break off. A kerion occurs when the affected areas become swollen and tender (**Figure 10.11**).
- **Tinea cruris:** this forms the inguinal (crural) folds. It is much more common in men with concomitant tinea pedis, particularly in those who sweat copiously. It occurs frequently in obese and diabetic individuals.
- **Dermatophyte onychomycosis:** toenails are discoloured and may be white or brown/yellowish in colour.

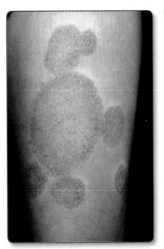

Figure 10.10 Tinea corporis.

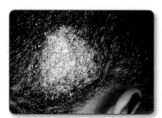

Figure 10.11 Tinea capitis.

Investigation

Investigations include the following.

- Skin scrapings, scalp brushings and nail clippings are essential investigations
- Microscopy and culture can be used to identify organisms
- Potassium hydroxide (KOH) can be added to skin scrapings from the lesions and examined under the microscope; the presence of hyphae in the specimen confirms dermatophyte infection.

Treatment

Topical antifungal creams can be used for treatment in the first instance. Infections refractory to topical treatment or severe tinea infection require treatment with oral terbinafine or griseofulvin. The duration and dose of medication vary according to patient age and affected site. A 3-month course of terbinafine is usually required in adults for dermatophyte onychomycosis of the fingernails and up to 9 months for the toenails.

Candida spp.

This yeast is a normal part of the flora of the gastrointestinal and genitourinary tracts. Disease may occur in the mucous membranes or nails. Invasive infections and certain mucocutaneous infections are signs of immunosuppression.

Clinical features

Oral candidiasis ('thrush')

Inflammatory change occurs

Clinical insight

Dermatophytes commonly cause toenail onychomycosis, and yeasts fingernail onychomycosis.

in the oropharynx often with associated white exudate and plaques (**Figure 10.12**).

Vulvovaginitis The main symptoms are itching and white discharge. There are inflammatory changes on the vulva and patients may report dysuria or dyspareunia. Antibiotic use, corticosteroid use and diabetes are all risk factors for this condition.

Balinitis Patients report pain and itch on the penis, and white patches may be present too. Infection may spread to adjacent tissues.

Candidal intertrigo Infection is in the inguinal folds, axillae, scrotum, inframammary folds, intergluteal folds or abdominal folds. Erythematous macerated plaques and erosions, with peripheral scaling and satellite erythematous papules or pustules, appear (**Figure 10.13**).

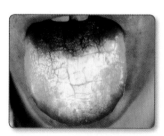

Figure 10.12 Oral candidiasis.

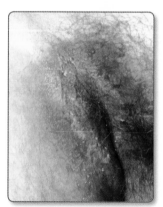

Figure 10.13 Candidal intertrigo.

Obesity, hyperhidrosis, incontinence, diabetes, cortico-steroid therapy, immunosuppressant therapy and impaired T-cell-mediated immunity are all risk factors for this.

Systemic infection Immunocompromised patients are at risk of candidaemia. These patients may develop inflammatory pustules or nodules at any skin site due to haematogenous spread.

Investigations
Investigations include:
- microbiology swabs showing budding yeasts on Gram stain and culture of *Candida* spp.
- KOH microscopy showing pseudohyphae
- blood cultures, swabs and skin biopsy, which may be per-formed in suspected cases of systemic candidiasis with skin involvement

Treatment
Treatment is with either a topical or a systemic agent.
- **Topical agents:** nystatin, miconazole, clotrimazole or ketoconazole may be used for intertrigo. Low-dose cor-ticosteroid is present in some agents to help reduce pain and pruritus
- **Systemic agents:** oral or intravenous fluconazole and itra-conazole are the main agents used

Malassezia spp.
Malassezia is a yeast that is a commensal in human skin.

Clinical features
These include the following.
- **Seborrhoeic dermatitis:** this is partly secondary to over-growth of *Malassezia furfur*.
- **Pityriasis versicolor:** patients develop hypo- or hyperpigment-ed scaly erythematous macules and patches (**Figure 10.14**). The rash occurs on the upper trunk and proximal arms.

Differential diagnoses include seborrhoeic dermatitis, pityriasis rosea, erythrasma, secondary syphilis, vitiligo and mycosis fungoides.

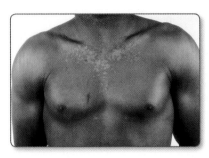

Figure 10.14 Pityriasis versicolor.

Investigations

Examination of the rash with Wood's lamp reveals yellow–green fluorescence in around 40% of cases. KOH preparation shows hyphae and yeast cells ('spaghetti and meatballs').

Treatment

For seborrhoeic dermatitis, see page 129.

Pityriasis versicolor

Topical Ketoconazole 2% shampoo used three times a week to scalp and skin may be an effective treatment. Ketoconazole cream 2% may also be added to the regimen.
Systemic Itraconazole and fluconazole may be used in severe or unresponsive disease.

Moulds

Moulds are fungi present in indoor and outdoor environments. Infections occur in immunosuppressed patients. Infection is often systemic and secondary to species such as *Aspergillus* and *Fusarium*.

Cutaneous infection usually consists of abscesses.

10.5 Mycobacterial infections

Cutaneous tuberculosis

Infection with *Mycobacterium tuberculosis* may be due to primary inoculation of the organism into the skin or disseminated systemic infection.

Atypical mycobacteria

These organisms include *Myocbacterium chelonae* and *M. abscessus*, which are ubiquitous in the environment, so infection can occur in immunocompetent individuals. There is a risk of transmission through contaminated instruments in procedures such as tattooing, liposuction and breast implants.

Clinical features

These include:

- papules, verrucous plaques and suppurative nodules
- lesions which are usually unilateral and spread from distal to proximal in the distribution of the lymphatics (spirotrichoid spread)

Investigations

These include:

- skin biopsy: for haematoxylin and eosin (H&E) staining and mycobacterial culture
- PCR: skin biopsy can be sent for PCR studies to characterise organisms

Treatment

Multidrug therapy is used to treat cutaneous TB and atypical mycobacterial infections. Agents include isoniazid, rifampicin, pyrazinamide and ethambutol.

Leprosy (Hansen's disease)

This is caused by *Mycobacterium leprae*; it affects the nerves and skin. It occurs more commonly in India, South-East Asia and Brazil.

Clinical features

These include:

- hypopigmented or erythematous patches on the skin (**Figure 10.15**)
- tender, enlarged peripheral nerves with neuropathy
- swellings on the earlobes/face, with the so-called 'leonine facies'

Investigations

A skin biopsy and PCR should be performed.

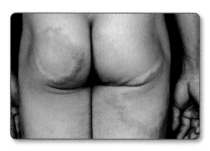

Figure 10.15 Leprosy.

Treatment

Multidrug therapy is used to treat leprosy. Agents commonly used together are dapsone, rifampicin and clofazimine. Treatment continues for 6–12 months.

10.6 Infestations

Scabies

This is an intensely itchy eruption caused by the mite *Sarcoptes scabiei*. The mite is transmitted by direct person-to-person contact. In adults the route of transmission is usually sexual.

Differential diagnoses include severe atopic eczema, tinea corporis, papular urticaria and seborrhoeic dermatitis.

Clinical features

These are as follows.

- Intense pruritus is worst at night; symptoms start between 3 and 6 weeks after infestation
- Patients develop erythematous papules that may have haemorrhagic crusts
- Typically these papules are in the finger webs, flexor aspects of the wrist, elbows, axillae, ears, nipples, umbilicus and genitals
- The scalp and face may be involved in children, the elderly and immunocompromised individuals
- The pathognomonic sign in scabies is the burrow. It is a thin erythematous or greyish line in affected sites (**Figure 10.16**)

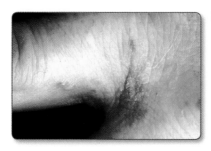

Figure 10.16 Scabies.

- In an immunocompetent individual the number of mites declines after 2–3 weeks
- Crusted scabies occurs in immunocompromised individuals Patients have scaly, thickened and crusted skin changes.

Investigations

Microscopy is performed on skin scrapings, usually taken from the finger web spaces. The mite and eggs should be visible in cases of scabies and can be skilfully removed using the tip of a green needle.

Treatment

Treatment is with two applications of permethrin 5% cream 7 days apart. It should be left in place for 8–12 hours and washed off. Adults should use a 30-g tube for one treatment. If permethrin treatment is not effective, oral ivermectin can be given, although this should be under specialist supervision.

Pediculosis (lice)

Lice are wingless insects that commonly cause infestation on the head or body. Head lice most commonly affect children and their presence is independent of hygiene or socioeconomic status. Body lice are associated with poor personal hygiene, poverty and communal sleeping arrangements.

Clinical features

Pediculosis capitis Patients are relatively asymptomatic even in the presence of a large number of lice. After 2–6 weeks pruritus may occur, with erythema on the posterior neck and ears. Nits and lice can be found adherent to hairs.

Pediculosis corporis Patients are very itchy and usually have erythematous macules, papules and excoriation on their skin. The lice live on clothing, so no nits or lice are found on the body but may be found in clothing seams.

Treatment

Pediculosis capititis This should be with two applications of permethrin rinse 1% for 10 min before washing off. Patient should have two treatments 7 days apart.

Pediculosis corporis Ideally clothing and bedding should be incinerated. If this is not possible it must be washed at high temperature (>130°C). Topical permethrin 5% cream may be used in a similar regimen to that used to treat scabies.

Systemic diseases

Systemic diseases often involve the skin; in many cases the skin signs are what prompt investigation that reveals the underlying systemic disease. Clinicians need to be able to recognise cutaneous signs associated with systemic diseases and understand the key investigations required.

11.1 Clinical scenario

A 28-year-old woman presents to her general practitioner with a 4-day history of painful red 'lumps' on her lower legs. The severity of the pain is such that she cannot walk unaided. This is the second episode that she has had over the past 6 months, presenting each time in the same way and each episode lasting 8 weeks. During the episodes the patient feels feverish with joint aches and fatigue.

The patient is normally well and takes only the oral contraceptive pill. Specifically there is no history of sore throat, cough, weight loss or diarrhoea during or between episodes.

On examination there are erythematous nodules on the pretibial skin of both legs (**Figure 11.1**). These are extremely tender to palpation.

Diagnostic approach

Recurrent painful nodules on the anterior surface of the lower legs of a young female patient are suggestive of panniculitis, most probably erythema nodosum (EN). It is important to seek a history of streptococcal infection, tuberculosis (TB), inflammatory bowel disease or trauma, all of which may precipitate EN.

Investigations

Most cases are idiopathic but it is important that any treatable or serious underlying cause be excluded. Investigate for streptococcal infection: throat swab, anti-streptococcal O titre; and stool examination for organisms of gastroenteritis. Chest

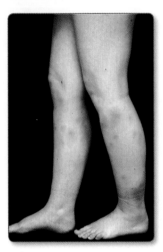

Figure 11.1 Erythema nodosum.

radiograph may reveal bilateral hilar lymphadenopathy in sarcoidosis or pulmonary infection of TB.

Management

Any treatable cause for EN should be addressed. In our clinical scenario the most likely cause is the contraceptive pill, and a trial off this medication may help. Most cases are self-limiting, so symptomatic relief of the pain is all that is required. Non-steroidal anti-inflammatory drugs (NSAIDs) are of most benefit for pain relief. Compression hosiery is of benefit.

The lesions heal without scarring.

11.2 Cutaneous vasculitis

Cutaneous vasculitis is the inflammation of the blood vessels of the skin; it may be primary or secondary to other diseases such as lupus. There is damage to the wall of the vessel by:

- direct injury from a bacterium or virus
- injury through activation of antibodies
- injury through activation of complement (proteins in the blood that attack infection and the vessel wall)

Causes of the disease may be classified into infective and non-infective (**Table 11.1**).

Infections	β-Haemolytic streptococci, mycobacteria, *Neisseria meningitidis*, hepatitis B and C, HIV, parvovirus B19, rickettsiae
Drugs	NSAIDs, anti-TNF agents, penicillins, propylthiouracil, minocycline
Inflammatory disease	Rheumatoid arthritis, systemic lupus erythematosus, inflammatory bowel disease
Malignancy	Multiple myeloma, haematological malignancy
Idiopathic	50% of cases

HIV, human immunodeficiency virus; NSAIDs, non-steroidal anti-inflammatory drugs; TNF, tumour necrosis factor.

Table 11.1 Causes of cutaneous vasculitis

Clinical features

Cutaneous vasculitis presents as a rash, usually on the lower limbs or distal aspect of the upper limbs. The size of the vessel affected gives rise to the clinical presentation seen.

> **Clinical insight**
>
> Patients with cutaneous vasculitis should always have a urine dipstick test performed and renal function investigated. Renal vasculitis can lead to rapidly progressive renal failure.

Vasculitis affecting the small vessels presents with a palpable purpura, typically affecting dependent sites. Medium-size vessel involvement presents with livedo reticularis, ulcers or subcutaneous nodules. **Table 11.2** details the clinical signs in cutaneous vasculitis.

Some patients will have systemic vasculitis as well as cutaneous disease. Presentations vary according to the organ involved (**Table 11.3**).

Investigations

For investigations, see **Table 11.4**.

Treatment

Once all the investigations to establish a possible cause have been completed, the

> **Clinical insight**
>
> Purpuric lesions in cutaneous vasculitis are usually palpable and affect sites of dependency.

Palpable purpura (**Figure 11.2**)	Non-blanchable purpuric lesions due to inflammation in venules and arterioles
Haemorrhagic bullae	Purpuric blisters filled with serosanguineous fluid due to tissue necrosis
Skin ulceration	Intense vasculitis compromises the blood supply to digits, leading to skin necrosis and ulceration
Livedo reticularis (**Figure 11.3**)	A reticulated (lacy) violaceous rash on the limbs. It may represent vasospasm or embolic phenomenon
Urticarial vasculitis	Erythematous and oedematous as in 'ordinary' urticaria. However, it persists for >24 hours and is painful rather than itchy

Table 11.2 Clinical signs in cutaneous vasculitis

Organ	Symptoms and signs
Cardiovascular	Chest pain, shortness of breath
Neurological	Headache, weakness, sensation change, altered behaviour, psychosis
Renal	Oedema, proteinuria, haematuria, hypertension
Musculoskeletal	Arthralgia, myalgia
General	Malaise, night sweats, fever, weight loss, hair loss, dry eyes and mouth
Gastrointestinal	Abdominal pain, per rectum bleeding, nausea, hepatomegaly, jaundice

Table 11.3 Clinical features of systemic cutaneous vasculitis

underlying cause should be treated. The extent of the vasculitis, in terms of systemic involvement, should be determined and treated according to the system type, but usually with corticosteroids.

In cases of isolated cutaneous disease the patient should be advised to rest and to elevate and compress swollen limbs to avoid progression to ulceration. NSAIDs are often used for pain relief.

Urine	Dipstick for blood and protein
Bloods	FBC, ESR, U&Es, glomerular filtration rate, protein:creatinine ratio, LFTs, serum calcium, ANCA, dsDNA, ENA, anticardiolipin antibodies, protein C and S levels, serum protein electrophoresis, HIV test, hepatitis serology
Skin biopsy	H&E stain, IMF, culture
Radiology	Chest radiograph
ANCA, anti-neutrophil cytoplasmic antibody; dsDNA, double-stranded DNA; ENA, extractable nuclear antigen; ESR, erythrocyte sedimentation rate; FBC, full blood count; H&E, haematoxylin and eosin; IMF, immunofluorescence; LFTs, liver function tests; U&Es, urea and electrolytes.	

Table 11.4 Investigations of cutaneous vasculitis

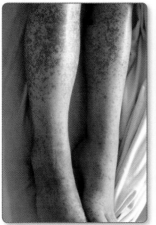

Figure 11.2 Palpable purpura.

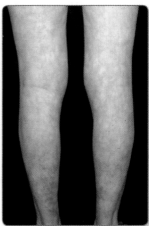

Figure 11.3 Livedo reticularis.

11.3 Panniculitis

This is inflammation of the subcutaneous fat, which typically presents as deep nodules on the lower legs. It may result from infection, malignancy or trauma, or be associated with an inflammatory disorder. Appropriate investigations are outlined in **Table 11.5**.

Aetiology

Inflammatory panniculitis

Erythema nodosum Classically this appears as tender erythematous nodules on the shins in young women. It may be associated with malaise and arthralgia. The causes include streptococcal infection, inflammatory bowel disease (IBD), sarcoidosis, the oral contraceptive pill, TB and Behçet's disease.

Lupus panniculitis Patients with systemic lupus erythematosus (SLE) develop erythematous nodules, which may develop on unusual sites such as the arms, shoulders, face and buttocks.

Cutaneous polyarteritis nodosa Patients present with tender nodules which may ulcerate and are associated with a livedoid rash, fever, malaise and arthralgia. The pathology is confined to the skin.

Erythema induratum ('nodular vasculitis') Patients are typically young women who develop nodules on the posterior aspects of their lower legs. Lesions ulcerate and are associated with TB or drugs.

Bloods	FBC, U&Es, LFTs, serum calcium, serum ACE, ANA, ENA, ANCA, ASOT, ESR, amylase, LDH, hepatitis B/C serology, TB screen
Radiology	Chest radiograph to exclude any evidence of TB, sarcoidosis or malignancy
Skin biopsy	Deep incisional biopsy required to analyse subcutaneous tissue

ACE, angiotensin-converting enzyme; ANA, antinuclear antibody; ANCA, anti-neutrophil cytoplasmic antibody; ASOT, anti-streptolysin O titre; ENA, extractable nuclear antigen; ESR, erythrocyte sedimentation rate; FBC, full blood count; LDH, lactate dehydrogenase; LFTs, liver function tests; TB, tuberculosis; U&Es, urea and electrolytes.

Table 11.5 Investigations in cases of panniculitis

Infectious panniculitis

Patients initially present with inflamed nodules and subsequently develop pustules and/or abscesses. This condition can be caused by any microorganism: bacteria, viruses, fungi or mycobacteria. It is caused by a direct extension of the infection into the skin. Immunosuppressed patients are more at risk of this phenomenon.

Malignancy-associated panniculitis

Subcutaneous, panniculitis-like, T-cell lymphoma Patients present with painless nodules on the extremities and/or trunk. There may be a history of fatigue, malaise and night sweats. Diagnosis of lymphoma is based on the histopathology and immunohistochemistry showing atypical lymphocytes.

Traumatic panniculitis

Direct trauma to the skin on the lower legs can lead to development of tender subcutaneous nodules. The condition can also occur at low temperatures.

Pancreatic panniculitis

Patients develop inflammatory nodules on the lower limbs, usually on the shins or around the ankles. Lesions appear suppurative and a brownish creamy liquid can drain from them. They are formed through lipolysis secondary to systemic release of pancreatic enzymes. The condition occurs in patients with pancreatic malignancy or severe pancreatitis.

Clinical features

Lesions frequently present on the lower limbs below the knee as deep nodules or plaques. There may be ulceration and erythema. The lesions are usually painful – deep nodules with plaques.

Investigations

For investigations, see **Table 11.5**.

Treatment

Panniculitis is treated by addressing the underlying cause. Adequate analgesia should be provided for the patient, with NSAIDs being the most effective. If ulceration occurs, compression therapy may be required.

11.4 Pyoderma gangrenosum

This rare and serious skin disorder is characterised by painful ulceration, more commonly seen on the lower legs and trunk. It is caused by unchecked neutrophil activity in the skin.

Pyoderma gangrenosum (PG) is most commonly found in association with:
- inflammatory bowel disease
- haematological disease including immunoglobulin (Ig)A monoclonal gammopathy, leukaemia, myeloma, myelodysplasia, lymphoma and polycythaemia vera
- rheumatoid arthritis, seronegative arthritis, ankylosing spondylitis

Differential diagnoses include vascular occlusion, cutaneous infection, a drug reaction and venous disease.

Clinical features

The initial lesion is a tender papule or pustule, which may have developed at the site of trauma (biopsy, insect bite). This rapidly enlarges and forms a cutaneous ulcer with a violaceous undermined edge (**Figure 11.4**). A crateriform lesion can appear within 48 hours. This then follows one of two courses:
1 rapid progression with systemic illness, fever and pain
2 indolent, with spontaneous healing at one site, and progression of a new lesion at another

Investigations

Investigations should be aimed at establishing the underlying cause of PG (**Table 11.6**).

An incisional skin biopsy may be performed to exclude other disorders, but some clinicians avoid this because of the risk of inducing further PG lesions (pathergy).

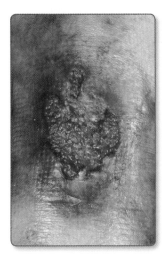

Figure 11.4 Pyoderma gangrenosum.

Tests	Description
Bloods	FBC, U&Es, LFTs, ANA, ANCA, hepatitis B and C, rheumatoid factor, electrophoresis, ESR
Radiology	Chest radiograph to exclude infection
Colonoscopy	Exclude inflammatory bowel disease

ANA, antinuclear antibody; ANCA, anti-neutrophil cytoplasmic antibody; ENA, extractable nuclear antigen; ESR, erythrocyte sedimentation rate; FBC, full blood count; LFTs, liver function tests; U&Es, urea and electrolytes.

Table 11.6 Investigations for pyoderma gangrenosum

Treatment

All patients should be given adequate analgesia. Wounds should be cared for in a specialist centre. Highly absorbent wound dressings should be used together with a thick barrier ointment and compression therapy where possible.

Mild disease may respond to topical steroid or intralesional steroid therapy. More extensive disease requires systemic agents, e.g. corticosteroids, ciclosporin or dapsone. The anti-tumour necrosis factor (TNF) agents, including infliximab and adalimumab, have been used with some success.

11.5 Calciphylaxis

This condition is characterised by ischaemia and skin necrosis due to calcification of arterioles deep within the skin. Most commonly it occurs in patients with end-stage renal disease who require dialysis. It is associated with a high mortality, usually secondary to infection from the skin ulceration. Differential diagnoses include a thromboembolic event (e.g. atherosclerosis) or skin necrosis caused by warfarin.

Clinical features

There may be associated livedo reticularis due to ischaemia in blood vessels to the skin. The disease starts with a purple mottling of the skin, usually on the lower limb or abdomen; bleeding then occurs within the mottling, and large areas of black crust appear on the skin due to skin necrosis (**Figure 11.5**). There is often white stellate-shaped scars within the area. Affected areas are extremely painful.

Investigations

This diagnosis is mainly a clinical one. Blood tests commonly show impaired renal function, and may show elevated parathyroid hormone. An incisional biopsy can help determine the diagnosis, but it should be avoided in patients who have systemic sepsis.

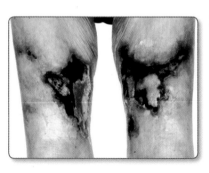

Figure 11.5 Calciphylaxis.

Treatment

Analgesia (often opiates) is required for all patients. Calcium and phosphate levels should be normalised and, in patients undergoing dialysis, the dialysate can be changed to one with a lower calcium concentration. Oxygen therapy to reduce ischaemia (15 L for 2 hours per day) can be initiated. Intravenous sodium thiosulphate has been used to good effect. Input from a dermatological nurse should occur for wound care to debride necrotic areas and keep the wound clean.

11.6 Rheumatic disease

Rheumatic diseases are primarily disorders of the joints, but these diseases, and many of the medications used to treat them, can affect the skin. Some cutaneous features are associated with rheumatological disease and others are pathognomonic for it. When treating patients with known rheumatic diseases it is important to note the skin symptoms and signs.

Raynaud's phenomenon

This is characterised by distinct colour changes of the skin on the digits. Classically it occurs in response to cold temperatures, although it may also be induced by emotional stress. The colour change is as follows:

White/pallor → blue/cyanosis → red/erythema (**Figure 11.6**).

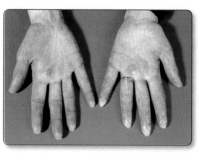

Figure 11.6 Raynaud's phenomenon.

The phenomenon is caused by abnormal vasoconstriction of digital arteries and cutaneous arterioles. It may occur in isolation (primary Raynaud's phenomenon [RP]) or as a result of another condition, e.g. systemic lupus erythematosus (SLE), scleroderma or dermatomyositis (secondary RP).

Systemic lupus erythematosus

This multisystem disease involves the skin in over 80% of cases. The severity of cutaneous involvement is variable. Important investigations to perform are outlined in **Table 11.7**.

Clinical features

Mucocutaneous features The most common manifestation of acute SLE is an erythematous, oedematous, butterfly rash (**Figure 11.7**), which affects the nose and cheeks but spares the nasolabial folds. It is a photosensitive rash that is worse after sun exposure. The rash lasts a few days after sun exposure and is often mistaken for sunburn. Differential diagnoses for the butterfly rash include rosacea, drug-induced rash and seborrhoeic dermatitis.

Associated cutaneous and mucocutaneous features The associated features are:
- alopecia
- episcleritis, scleritis, anterior uveitis
- oral ulceration

Tests	Description
Bloods	FBC, U&Es, LFTs, ANA, ENA, ANCA, anti-phospholipid antibodies, complement, ESR, CK
Urine	Dipstick, protein:creatinine ratio
Skin biopsy	H&E stain, IMF

ANA, antinuclear antibody; ANCA, anti-neutrophil cytoplasmic antibody; CK, creatine kinase; DLE, discoid lupus erythematosus; ENA, extractable nuclear antigen; ESR, erythrocyte sedimentation rate; FBC, full blood count; H&E, haematoxylin and eosin; IMF, immunofluorescence; LFTs, liver function tests; SCLE, acute cutaneous lupus erythematosus; SLE, systemic lupus erythematosus; U&Es, urea and electrolytes.

Table 11.7 Investigations for SLE/DLE/SCLE

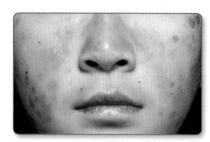

Figure 11.7 Butterfly rash of systemic lupus erythematosus.

- bullous vasculitis
- panniculitis known as lupus profundus; patients develop painful panniculitic lesions during flares of SLE

Systemic features

During a flare of SLE, patients may have fatigue, myalgia, arthralgia, weight loss, lymphadenopathy and fever. The systemic features are summarised in **Table 11.8**.

Treatment

Patients should:
- avoid exacerbating drugs: tetracyclines, sulfonamides and procainamide
- use strict photoprotection
- patients who may require vitamin D replacement if deficient
- topical corticosteroids and intralesional steroids to any lesions refractory to topical therapy

Topical calcineurin inhibitors may be used in place of topical corticosteroids. If topical therapies are ineffective, systemic treatment with antimalarial therapy (hydroxychloroquine) should be used.

Patients with SLE are usually treated with systemic therapies such as glucocorticoids, immunosuppression with cyclophosphamide or ciclosporin, or the B-cell-depletion agents rituximab and beliumumab.

> **Clinical insight**
>
> The incidence of congenital heart block in anti-Ro-positive women with SLE is 1–2% and 10 times higher for subsequent pregnancies. Increased ultrasound surveillance is advocated from week 16 of gestation.

System	Features
Cardiovascular	Libman–Sacks endocarditis Myocarditis Pericardial effusion
Respiratory	Pleural effusion Interstitial lung disease Recurrent DVT and/or PE pulmonary hypertension
Gastrointestinal	Vasculitis – can lead to colitis and pancreatitis
Nervous	Headache Delirium Psychosis Polyneuropathy Multiple cranial nerve palsies
Renal	Glomerulonephritis Proteinuria Haematuria Renal impairment/failure
Musculoskeletal	Migratory oligoarthritis Myalgia
Haematological	Anaemia of chronic disease Leukopenia Thrombophilia
Female reproductive	Recurrent miscarriage Risk of neonatal lupus and congenital heart block if positive for the Ro or La antibody

DVT, deep vein thrombosis; PE, pulmonary embolism.

Table 11.8 Systemic features of systemic lupus erythematosus (SLE)

Discoid lupus erythematosus

This is a chronic, photosensitive, skin eruption that heals with scarring. Patients with discoid lupus erythematosus (DLE) have an approximately 5% risk of having SLE or developing it. Patients with widespread discoid lesions are thought to be at higher risk of developing SLE.

Differential diagnoses include tinea faciei, sarcoidosis, cutaneous TB ('lupus vulgaris') and lymphoproliferative disorders of the skin.

Clinical features

Discoid lupus erythematosus is characterised by discrete, erythematous, infiltrated, perifollicular, scaly plaques (**Figure 11.8**). The rash destroys hair follicles, and leads to scarring and alopecia. The sites exposed to ultraviolet (UV) are those classically involved, i.e. the cheeks, nose, ears and back of hands.

Investigation and management

A biopsy is performed to confirm the diagnosis. Strict photoprotection is recommended for all patients, with vitamin D supplementation if required. The main aim of treatment is to limit the scarring because the sites involved are functionally and cosmetically sensitive. Potent topical corticosteroids are used. If systemic treatment is required, hydroxychloroquine is the first-line agent. Some patients will require advice on cosmetic camouflage.

Subacute cutaneous lupus erythematosus

About 50% of patients with subacute cutaneous lupus erythematosus (SCLE) have SLE. It can be drug induced, and patients with SCLE should avoid the medications listed in **Table 11.9**.

Differential diagnoses include psoriasis vulgaris, tinea corporis, mycosis fungoides, erythema multiforme and dermatomyositis.

Clinical features

Early lesions are scaly papules, which become annular and often polycyclic. The edge of the annular lesions is erythematous and

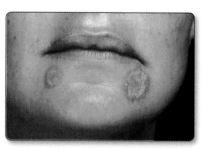

Figure 11.8 Discoid lupus erythematosus.

Types of lupus	Drugs
SLE	Procainamide, hydralazine, diltiazem, hydrochlorthiazide, penicillamine, isoniazid, infliximab, etanercept, minocycline
SCLE	Hydrochlorthiazide, diltiazem, ACE inhibitors, anti-TNF-α agents, PPIs, lamotrigine, terbinafine

ACE, angiotensin-converting enzyme; PPI, proton pump inhibitor; SCLE, subacute cutaneous lupus erythematosus; SLE, systemic lupus erythematosus; TNF, tumour necrosis factor.

Table 11.9 Drugs that may induce lupus erythematosus

crusted. The rash most commonly affects the upper chest, neck, shoulders and neck, and is extremely photosensitive.

Treatment
The treatment for SCLE is the same as the that for SLE (see page 189).

Dermatomyositis
Dermatomyositis (DM) is an idiopathic inflammatory myopathy characterised by inflammation of the muscles and the skin, resulting in proximal weakness, myositis and cutaneous disease.

Clinical features
Patients usually have proximal muscle weakness and associated cutaneous signs (**Figure 11.9**):
- heliotrope rash with periorbital oedema
- Gottron's papules, which are violaceous papules over the metacarpophalangeal and interphalangeal joints
- facial erythema and oedema
- photodistributed rash classically like a shawl on the shoulders or on the upper chest in the shape of a V
- periungal erythema and cuticle overgrowth
- cutaneous ulceration in some cases
- Raynaud's phenomenon and panniculitis possibly common

There may be the following associated systemic features:
- **respiratory:** interstitial lung disease
- **gastrointestinal:** dysphagia, regurgitation due to muscle weakness, risk of aspirational pneumonia

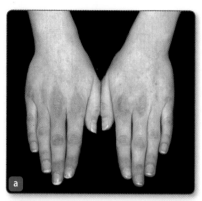

Figure 11.9 Cutaneous signs of dermatomyositis.

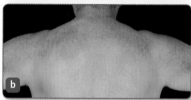

- **cardiac:** myocarditis and dysrhythmia described
- **malignancy:** in some cases DM may be triggered by an underlying malignancy.

Investigations

For the investigations of DM see **Table 11.10**.

Treatment

The treatment for DM is the same as the treatment for SLE (see page 189).

Systemic sclerosis (scleroderma)

Scleroderma itself means hardening of the skin. Localised scleroderma is known as morphea and is not associated with systemic complications. Systemic sclerosis (SSc) most commonly occurs in women and presents around the age of 40. Systemic disease can be divided into two types: limited cutaneous SSc and diffuse cutaneous SSc.

Tests	Description
Bloods	FBC, U&Es, LFTs, CK, LDH, AST, ALT, ESR, ANA, ENA, myositis-specific antibodies
Skin biopsy	H&E stain, IMF
EMG	Changes of inflammatory myopathy
MRI	Myositis can be seen on MRI – thighs and upper arms are usually imaged.
Muscle biopsy	Injury to myofibres identified

ALT, alanine aminotransferase; ANA, antinuclear antibody; AST, aspartate aminotransferase; CK, creatine kinase; ENA, extractable nuclear antigen; FBC, full blood count; H&E, haematoxylin and eosin; IMF, immunofluorescence; LDH, lactate dehydrogenase; LFTs, liver function tests; U&Es, urea and electrolytes.

Table 11.10 Investigations in dermatomyositis

Clinical features

Cutaneous features of systemic sclerosis The clinical features include:

- scleroderma: hardening of the skin – usually swollen and itchy before hardening occurs
- sclerodactyly: characteristic tapering of the fingertips (**Figure 11.10**)
- digital ulcers
- telangiectasia
- calcinosis: deposits of calcium in the skin (**Figure 11.11**)
- Raynaud's phenomenon

Limited cutaneous SSc This is limited to the hands, forearms, neck and face. Patients present with **CREST** syndrome – **c**alcinosis, **R**aynaud's phenomenon, o**e**sophageal dysmotility, **s**clerodactyly and **t**elangiectasia.

Those with a long history of limited cutaneous SSc may develop interstitial lung disease, pulmonary hypertension and gastrointestinal (GI) disease. Renal disease rarely occurs. The majority (60%) are positive for the anti-centromere antibody.

Diffuse cutaneous SSc Patients with diffuse cutaneous SSc have sclerotic skin on their upper arms, shoulders, chest and

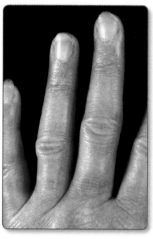

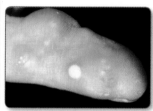

Figure 11.10 Sclerodactyly.   **Figure 11.11** Calcinosis.

abdomen. They develop early interstitial lung, renal, GI and myocardial disease. Patients are positive for the anti-SCL-70 antibody in around 40% of cases.

Complications The systemic complications associated with SSc are:

- **respiratory:** interstitial lung disease, pulmonary hypertension, increased risk of lung cancer
- **cardiovascular:** pericarditis, pericardial effusion, myocardial fibrosis and heart failure
- **gastrointestinal:** gastro-oesophageal reflux, oesophagitis and oesophageal stricture formation; chronic reflux may lead to Barrett's oesophagus
- **renal:** renal impairment that progresses to renal failure

Investigations

Scleroderma is a clinical diagnosis but certain investigations may be helpful (**Table 11.11**).

Treatment

Treatment options for scleroderma include superpotent topical steroids, systemic treatment such as methotrexate or UVA

Tests	Description
Bloods	FBC, U&Es, LFTs, ANA, ENA, anti-centromere antibody, anti Scl-70
Skin biopsy	H&E stain
Imaging	High-resolution CT of the chest Barium swallow
Endoscopy	OGD
Cardiorespiratory	Transthoracic echo, respiratory function tests

ANA, antinuclear antibody; CT, computerised tomography; ENA, extractable nuclear antigen; FBC, full blood count; H&E, haematoxylin and eosin; LFTs, liver function tests; OGD, oesophagogastroduodenoscopy; U&Es, urea and electrolytes.

Table 11.11 Investigations in scleroderma

phototherapy. Vasodilators such as calcium channel blockers, phosphodiesterase type 5 (PDE5) inhibitors and/or prostacyclin infusions are used to treat Raynaud's phenomenon.

Renal and pulmonary physicians should be closely involved in controlling systemic and pulmonary hypertension.

Rheumatoid arthritis

Rheumatoid arthritis (RA) is an inflammatory disorder primarily involving the joints. It is more common in women and white people, with a peak onset around the age of 60 years, although it can occur at any age. Without appropriate treatment it is a cause of significant morbidity and mortality.

Differential diagnoses include viral polyarthritis, reactive arthritis, psoriatic arthritis, gout and pseudogout, and rarely Lyme arthritis.

Cutaneous features of RA

Patients may develop a wide array of skin changes in RA:

- non-specific skin changes: secondary to glucocorticoids – bruising, atrophy, brittle nails, palmar erythema
- rheumatoid nodules: skin-coloured nodules usually occurring on the extensor surfaces of the arms; they are usually firm and painless

- Raynaud's phenomenon
- neutrophilic dermatoses: Sweet's syndrome
- rheumatoid vasculitis: blood vessels damaged by RA; causes petechiae, nailfold infarct, ulceration

Treatment

Treatment for the skin disease is specific for each disorder. Rheumatoid nodules usually need no treatment, although intralesional steroids or surgical excision could be considered for debilitating lesions. Associated inflammatory disorders usually require specialist intervention.

Behçet's disease

This is a systemic vasculitis characterised by recurrent oral and genital ulceration. It is more common in patients

> **Clinical insight**
>
> Pathergy testing shows a papulopustular lesion that appears 48 hours after the skin prick with a 20-gauge needle

from Mediterranean and eastern Asian countries, and typically affects people aged 20–40 years.

Differential diagnoses include herpes simplex infection, benign aphthous ulcers, IBD and SLE.

Clinical features

There is recurrence of painful **oral aphthous ulcers** up to 2 cm in size. Ulcers are well defined with an erythematous edge. They occur inside the mouth and may preclude eating. Oral ulceration must occur more than three times a year to fulfil the diagnostic criteria for Behçet's disease. **Genital ulcers** are similar in appearance to oral ones. They are found on the scrotum in men and the vulva in women. These ulcers leave scarring on resolution. This scarring is a unique feature of Behçet's disease.

In addition there may be an acneiform eruption with a papulopustular and/or nodular component, a panniculitis, usually erythema nodosum, or superficial thrombophlebitis.

The clinical features of extracutaneous disease include:

- neurological disease: central nervous system (CNS) vasculitis, which may lead to vascular thrombosis, seizures, aseptic meningitis and personality change

- arthritis: in about 50% of patients with an intermittent large joint arthritis (knee, ankle, wrist)
- vascular symptoms: recurrent DVT, which may be a presenting feature; arterial vasculitis is less common and can affect coronary arteries and pulmonary arteries, leading to myocardial infarction and haemoptysis
- GI symptoms: ulceration which may occur at any point in the GI tract and lead to nausea, abdominal pain and/or diarrhoea
- eye symptoms: uveitis and retinal vasculitis, which may lead to loss of sight

Investigations

The diagnosis can be made in the absence of systemic disease. Patients must have recurrent oral ulceration (more than three times a year) and two of:

- recurrent genital ulceration
- eye lesions
- skin lesions
- positive pathergy test

No specific investigations are required to make a diagnosis of Behçet's disease. Bloods may show elevated inflammatory markers and pathergy testing may be useful.

Treatment

This should be initiated under specialist control and is usually one of the following: systemic corticosteroids, colchicine, azathioprine, cyclophosphamide, ciclosporin or mycophenolate mofetil. Anti-TNF-α agents have also been used.

Reactive arthritis

Also known as Reiter's syndrome, this is a post-infectious reactive arthritis with skin changes. It is associated with HIV and HLA-B27, and tends to occur in younger people. Differential diagnoses include IBD, poststreptococcal arthritis and disseminated gonococcal infection.

Clinical features

The symptoms occur about 4–6 weeks after infection with one of the organisms shown in **Table 11.12**. These organisms

Enteric	*Salmonella, Shigella, Campylobacter* spp., and *Clostridium difficile*
Genital	*Chlamydia trachomatis*
Retrovirus	HIV

Table 11.12 Causative organisms in Reiter's syndrome

cause urinary tract or GI infections, but patients may have an asymptomatic infection.

The symptoms include fever and malaise. There are hyperkeratotic lesions on the palms and soles (**Figure 11.12**), together with subungal hyperkeratosis, onycholysis and periungal erythema. There is usually oral ulceration and an asymmetrical oligoarthritis often affects the lower limbs. Enthesitis, i.e. swelling at the site of insertion of ligaments, most commonly affects the heels; dactylitis, conjunctivitis and anterior uveitis may be present.

Investigations

Acute phase reactants such as C-reactive protein (CRP) and erythrocyte sedimentation rate (ESR) will be elevated. Serology may show evidence of recent infection with one of the probable culprit organisms.

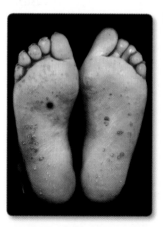

Figure 11.12 Reiter's syndrome.

Treatment

The skin changes are treated as plaques of psoriasis with topical steroids and salicylate preparations. Options for arthritis vary according to the severity of disease but include NSAIDs, oral and intra-articular glucocorticoids, sulfasalazine and methotrexate.

11.7 Haematological and oncological disease

Metastatic disease

Cutaneous metastases are relatively rare and associated with a poor prognosis.

Clinical features

Cutaneous metastases usually occur close to the location of the primary malignancy. Often metastases present as a firm, painless, erythematous nodule (**Figure 11.13**). Breast cancer is most likely to metastasise to the skin.

Investigations

Prompt skin biopsy is essential to establish the diagnosis.

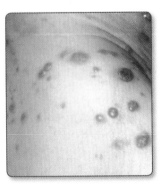

Figure 11.13 Cutaneous metastasis.

Treatment

Surgical excision, chemotherapy and radiotherapy are all options. The patient's oncology team must be involved in treatment decisions.

Cutaneous T-cell lymphoma

Mycosis fungoides (MF) is the most common type of cutaneous T-cell lymphoma (CTCL). It is a non-Hodgkin's lymphoma characterised by infiltration of the skin by clonal T cells. Systemic involvement occurs in more aggressive disease. Typically it affects adults aged >50 years.

Clinical features

Mycosis fungoides is often an indolent disease. For many decades before the diagnosis of MF, patients may have scaly, non-specific, skin disease which may be called 'parapsoriasis'. In its early stages MF mimics many benign dermatoses.

The presentation of MF is outlined in **Table 11.13**. It is important to note that patients usually do not progress through each stage.

Patch stage MF	Erythematous, scaly patches, up to 15 cm across, which may be pruritic. Classic sites of involvement are the buttocks and trunk. Patients may have only patch stage disease, and disease does not necessarily progress
Plaque stage MF	Patches become more infiltrated and oedematous
Tumour stage MF	Patients may go on to develop cutaneous nodules (tumours)
Erythrodermic MF	Patients may present with widespread erythroderma with signs of MF. If they present with just erythroderma a diagnosis of Sézary's syndrome should be considered
Sézary's syndrome	T-cell clones in the blood as well as in the skin. A small proportion of cases are associated with the human T-lymphotrophic viruses type 1 and 2 (HTLV-1, -2), which is common in Japan, the Caribbean and the Middle East

Table 11.13 Clinical presentation of mycosis fungoides (MF)

Investigations

Mycosis fungoides is diagnosed when a clonal T-cell population is identified in the skin. Key investigations in suspected cases of MF are:

- skin biopsy for haematoxylin and eosin (H&E) staining studies (looking for atypical lymphocytes) and T-cell rearrangement (looking for a T-cell clone)
- bloods including a count of Sézary's cells
- in some cases a lymph node biopsy

All cases should be sent to a specialist centre for assessment, investigation and staging.

Treatment

These diseases are rarely curable and the goal is to keep the disease under control while minimising the side effects of treatment. Early disease can be treated with topical corticosteroids, topical retinoids, topical chemotherapy, electron beam therapy or phototherapy. More advanced disease can be treated with agents such as systemic retinoids, methotrexate and interferon.

Prognosis is important to explain to patients. Those with very early stage 1A disease will have a normal life expectancy. Those with stage 2B have a median survival of 3.2 years. Those with stage 4A disease have a median survival of <1.5 years.

Paraneoplastic dermatoses

If any of the dermatoses below present (**Figure 11.14**) it is essential to obtain a thorough history and systems review, perform a full examination of systems, take bloods and request a chest radiograph. Other imaging should be requested according to the history and signs found.

Acanthosis nigricans

Patients present with velvety hyperpigmented plaques in the axillae and groins. Acanthosis nigricans is more commonly associated with obesity and insulin resistance; however, it can occur with the following malignancies: gastric carcinoma, hepatocellular carcinoma, and adenocarcinoma of the lung, ovary, kidney, pancreas, bladder, breast and endometrium.

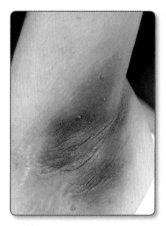

Figure 11.14 Acanthosis nigricans

Paraneoplastic pemphigus

Patients present with painful stomatitis and may have tense blisters on their body. The condition is associated with non-Hodgkin's lymphoma, chronic lymphocytic leukaemia and other lymphoproliferative disorders. It is diagnosed using serum sample showing anti-plakin antibodies.

Leser–Trélat sign

The sign is sudden onset of multiple seborrhoeic keratoses, some of which are on an inflammatory base. It is a sign of internal malignancy, most commonly GI, breast or lung cancer.

Palmar hyperkeratosis

Patients present with a yellowish thickening of the palms and soles, known as hyperkeratosis or tylosis. It is strongly associated with carcinoma of the oesophagus, breast, Hodgkin's lymphoma and leukaemia.

Necrolytic migratory erythema

This is a transient eczematous or psoriasiform rash which occurs around orifices, flexures and acral surfaces. Patients feel unwell and may have stomatitis, abdominal pain and diarrhoea. Classically it occurs with pancreatic tumours that secrete glucagon.

Necrolytic migratory erythema has also occurred with hepatocellular and lung cancer.

Erythema gyratum repens

This rash consists of concentric rings of erythematous plaques. The rash covers most of the patient's body and is extremely itchy. It is associated with lung, oesophageal and breast cancer.

Graft-versus-host disease

Graft-versus-host disease (GVHD) is a complication of an allogeneic stem cell transplantation. It occurs when immune cells from the donor (graft) recognise the recipient's host cells as foreign. An immune reaction is triggered and it can make the transplant recipient unwell. As well as mucosal and cutaneous symptoms, patients may also have GI symptoms, because a similar graft-versus-host reaction occurs in the gut and liver; the symptoms are anorexia, nausea, vomiting, abdominal pain and diarrhoea.

Clinical cutaneous features

The condition may be divided into categories according to time of onset after the stem cell transplantation (STC); this boundary is becoming blurred, however, with changes to transplantation regimens:
- acute GVHD (acute inflammatory skin changes) – occurs <100 days after STC
- chronic GVHD (chronic, fibrotic skin changes) – occurs >100 days after STC

  The morphology of the rash in GVHD is variable. Common forms encountered are:
- maculopapular
- eczematous
- lichenoid
- morphea-like
- poikilodermatous
- erythematous

Important differentials for this condition are a drug reaction or rash secondary to infection.

Investigations

A skin or GI tract biopsy is helpful in confirming the diagnosis. Histological changes reflect the morphology of the rash, e.g. lichenoid or morpheaform. Liver involvement is also relatively common and patients may have deranged liver function tests (LFTs).

Treatment

Treatment for mild GVHD is with topical corticosteroids and emollients. More severe forms of GVHD may require immunosuppression with agents such as prednisolone, ciclosporin, mycophenolate mofetil, phototherapy or photopheresis.

Sweet's syndrome

This is an acute febrile inflammatory disorder, associated with infection, IBD and RA. When the disease becomes chronic and recurrent, underlying haematological malignancy, particularly myelodysplasia, must be excluded. Differential diagnoses include systemic infection and necrotising fasciitis.

Clinical features

The patient is usually systemically unwell with a high fever and malaise. There is acute onset of erythematous, swollen papules, plaques or nodules, which can be widespread and are extremely painful.

Investigations

Patients have a markedly elevated white cell count, predominantly a neutrophilia, and elevated inflammatory markers. A septic screen will be negative. Skin biopsy from involved skin shows oedema and a florid neutrophilic infiltrate in the dermis.

Treatment

Topical corticosteroids can be used initially. In refractory cases systemic corticosteroids can be used.

11.8 Endocrine disease

Cutaneous signs occur in a number of endocrine disorders and often prove useful in making the diagnosis. The skin conditions usually resolve with treatment of the underlying disorder.

Diabetes

The following skin disorders can occur in diabetes:

- **Acanthosis nigricans** (see page 202).
- **Necrobiosis lipoidica:** there are yellow atrophic patches with an erythematous edge. They usually occur on the shins and occasionally ulcerate, and can be treated with intralesional triamcinolone.
- **Diabetic dermopathy:** patients present with brown macules and patches on the legs, which are thought to be caused by trauma. No specific treatment is required.
- **Neuropathic ulcers:** these most commonly occur on the legs and feet. Patients with sensory neuropathy develop ulcers at the site of pressure points, e.g. ball of the foot.
- **Granuloma annulare (GA):** this is a non-scaly, erythematous annular patch or plaque. If multiple lesions occur, it is called disseminated GA. GA is associated with diabetes and dys-lipidaemia (**Figure 11.15**).

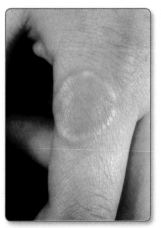

Figure 11.15 Granuloma annulare.

Feature	Hyperthyroidism	Hypothyroidism
Skin	• Palmar erythema and moist palms • Macular hyperpigmentation • Pruritus and urticaria • Pretibial myxoedema: Non-pitting scaly thickening of the skin on the pretibial skin often said to resemble an orange peel. May present as yellow brown indurated papules or nodules. 	• Dry, pale or yellow looking skin ('peaches and cream complexion') • Bruising due to capillary fragillty • Thickening of the skin on the palms and soles (keratoderma)
Hair	Fine, thin hair ± diffuse alopecia	Dull, brittle, alopecia of the lateral third of the eyebrow and alopecia areata common
Nails	Onycholysis, koilonychia and thyroid acropachy. Thyroid acropachy is clubbing and swelling of the fingers secondary to new periosteal bone formation.	Slow growing, brittle nails

Table 11.14 Features of thyroid disease

Thyroid disease

Thyroid function tests should be performed promptly if any of the signs detailed in **Table 11.14** are present.

Cushing's syndrome

Cushing's syndrome results from exposure to excess glucocorticoids. The causes include iatrogenic disease from prescribed corticosteroids, an adrenocorticotrophin hormone (ACTH)-secreting malignancy (classically lung cancer) or pituitary/adrenal tumours secreting ACTH (Cushing's disease).

It is of particular interest in dermatology because patients are frequently prescribed topical or systemic corticosteroids. It is essential that clinicians be aware of the features of Cushing's syndrome (**Figure 11.16**), which are:
- characteristic facial features: rounded face and full cheeks; possibly evidence of hirsutism and acne
- deposition of fat in the cervical vertebrae (buffalo hump)
- skin thinning (atrophy) and fragility; loss of subcutaneous fat and exposure of blood vessels
- easy bruising caused by stretching of fragile skin striae

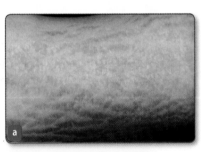

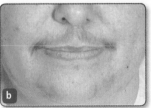

Figure 11.16 Cutaneous signs of Cushing's disease.

- hyperpigmentation
- fungal infection of the skin with dermatophytes or *Candida* spp.

The diagnosis can be confirmed with a urinary cortisol measurement and a dexamethasone suppression test.

Addison's disease

This disease occurs secondary to adrenal insufficiency. It may be secondary to autoimmune disease, infection within the adrenal gland or haemorrhage.

Patients feel unwell, are hypotensive, and have a low sodium, low glucose and high potassium. The following cutaneous features should alert the clinician:

- diffuse hyperpigmentation particularly in the palmar creases, mucous membranes, axillae and around the nipples
- hyperpigmentation on the mucous membranes, e.g. buccal mucosa
- increased incidence of autoimmune diseases

A short Synacthen test can be used to confirm the diagnosis.

Hyperlipidaemia

The cutaneous signs are associated with hyperlipidaemia and may indicate a genetically inherited disorder. All patients should have a full lipid profile performed, including total cholesterol, high-density lipoprotein (HDL), low-density lipoprotein (LDL) and triglycerides.

Xanthomas

These are yellow erythematous papules normally on the extensor surfaces (elbows, shins and hands). They are associated with elevated triglycerides (**Figure 11.17**).

Tendinous xanthomas

These are nodular deposits of lipid that occur on tendons. They are found most commonly on the Achilles tendon and the extensor tendons of the upper limbs. Familial hypercholesterolaemia and hypothyroidism are associated with them.

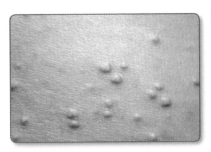

Figure 11.17 Xanthoma.

Plane xanthomas

These are yellowish macules, papules, patches and plaques that are well circumscribed and may occur anywhere on the body. They are strongly associated with familial hypercholesterolaemia and primary biliary cirrhosis.

Xanthelasma

This is plane xanthomas occurring on the skin of the eyelids. Interestingly only 50% of patients with xanthelasma have no underlying lipid disorder.

11.9 Gastrointestinal disease

Many diseases of the GI tract have dermatological manifestations; the signs seen in the skin can alert the physician to underlying disease or a flare of a known disease.

Inflammatory bowel disease

Both Crohn's disease and ulcerative colitis have dermatological findings in up to 40% of cases. The most common skin findings are:

- **fissures:** perianal fissures; treatment with a botulinum toxin injection or topical nitroglycerin
- **oral lesions:** aphthous ulceration, angular cheilitits (corner of the mouth inflammation); treatment with topical corticosteroids
- pyoderma gangrenosum: see page 184
- erythema nodosum

Coeliac disease

This is associated with a blistering disorder called dermatitis herpetiformis (see page 144).

Diseases associated with GI bleeding

Hereditary haemorrhagic telangiectasia

Patients frequently have telangiectasia on the skin and buccal mucosa (**Figure 11.18**). They may present with epistaxis and upper GI haemorrhage. Affected individuals have to be screened for arteriovenous malformations, especially in the lung, brain and liver.

Peutz–Jeghers syndrome

Patients present with pigmented macules on the lips and occasionally on the palms. This is an autosomal dominant disorder in which there are polyps throughout the GI tract that may bleed. There is an increased risk of bowel cancer.

Liver disease

Cutaneous signs of liver cirrhosis are: leukonychia, palmar erythema, jaundice, gynaecomastia and excoriation (due to intense pruritus).

Patients with hepatitis B or C may have:
- lichen planus with marked oral disease
- vasculitis secondary to cryoglobulins
- urticarial vasculitis
- porphyria cutanea tarda

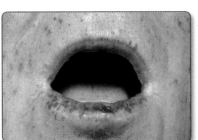

Figure 11.18 Hereditary haemorrhagic telangiectasia.

Patients with primary biliary cirrhosis may have severe cholestasis and develop planar xanthomas, especially on the palms.

11.10 Pulmonary disease

Sarcoidosis

This is a multisystem disorder of unknown aetiology characterised by the presence of granulomas. Typically it presents with pulmonary involvement and commonly affects the skin, eyes and joints. However, in some cases it affects only the skin. It is more common in those of African–Caribbean origin.

There is a highly variable pattern of presentation and organ involvement. Up to half of all cases are asymptomatic and diagnosed on a routine chest radiograph. Of patients 10–30% will have a chronic progressive pattern. Patients may have a fever, night sweats and weight loss. There is lung involvement in almost all cases, usually interstitial lung disease, presenting with chest discomfort and a dry cough. There is commonly eye involvement. There may be polyarthralgia or nerve palsies.

Clinical features of cutaneous sarcoid

These are the following:

- Cutaneous sarcoidosis most commonly presents as erythematous or red–brown papules or plaques that are flat topped (**Figure 11.19**).
- Lesions most commonly occur on the face, head, neck and upper trunk. Classic sites of involvement are the eyelids, nasal alae, forehead and sites of previous trauma (e.g. scars or tattoos).

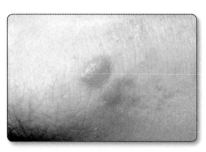

Figure 11.19 Cutaneous sarcoidosis.

- Occasionally lesions have associated hypopigmentation, ulcerate or appear like rosacea or morphea.
- Patients can present with erythema nodosum.
- Lupus pernio is a type of cutaneous sarcoid in which a clinically infiltrative papulonodular eruption affects the nose, ears and cheeks. It has a strong association with chronic pulmonary sarcoid.

Investigations

Skin biopsy is the investigation of choice to confirm a diagnosis of cutaneous sarcoidosis. It reveals 'naked' granulomas within the dermis.

Other key investigations are serum angiotensin-converting enzyme (ACE), full blood count, serum calcium and chest radiograph. If there is evidence of sarcoidosis, pulmonary function tests and high-resolution CT should be considered.

Treatment

Systemic corticosteroids and immunosuppressants are usually required.

Yellow nail syndrome

This is associated with a chronic suppurative lung disease such as bronchiectasis or chronic bronchitis.

Clinical features

Patients may describe cessation of nail growth followed by thickening of the nails. The cuticle disappears and there is yellow–green discoloration of the nail (**Figure 11.20**). Often all 20 nails are involved, with lymphoedema of periungal skin.

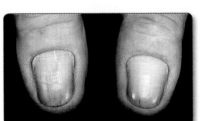

Figure 11.20 Yellow nail syndrome.

Treatment

Patients should be seen by a respiratory physician to treat their lung disease. In some cases oral fluconazole or itraconazole can be helpful for nail changes. Vitamin E has also been used.

11.11 Nutritional disorders

Nutritional deficiencies can cause skin changes. Some of the most common signs are listed in **Table 11.15**.

Vitamin deficiency	Common signs
A	Follicular papules with a central keratotic plug (phrynoderma)
B1 (thiamine)	Glossitis (**Figure 11.21**)
B6 (pyridoxine)	Seborrhoeic dermatitis, glossitis, angular cheilitis, stomatitis
C	Perifollicular erythema/haemorrhage with corkscrew hairs and follicular hyperkeratosis. Patients may also have petechiae, ecchymosis and bleeding gums
K	Purpura

Table 11.15 Common signs of vitamin deficiencies

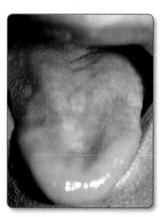

Figure 11.21 Glossitis.

Genital dermatoses

Genital dermatoses are associated with discomfort and embarrassment, and they affect body image and social functioning. Sensitivity about this necessitates tactful history taking and the use of a chaperone during examinations.

When taking the history it is important to discuss the patient's symptoms and the relationship of the symptoms to events, e.g. sexual intercourse or menstruation. Typical symptoms of a genital dermatosis include pruritus, genital pain, discharge from the penis/vagina and dyspareunia. Women should be asked about the pattern of their menstrual cycle and whether there has been a change to this. The patient's bowel habit and bladder function should be discussed. It is also important to ask if there are any associated oral symptoms. The dermatological and sexual history should be discussed along with any relevant psychosocial issues.

It is essential to be aware of genital anatomy and describe the location of lesions accurately (**Figure 12.1**).

Dermatoses in the genital area can arise due to the occurrence of:

- a common dermatosis (e.g. eczema) in the genital area

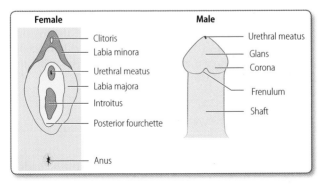

Figure 12.1 Genital anatomy.

- a specific genital inflammatory disease
- infection
- malignancy

12.1 Clinical scenario

Vulval rash and vaginal discharge

Presentation

A 50-year-old woman with diabetes mellitus, multiple sclerosis and myelodysplastic syndrome presents with a 2-week history of an itchy, burning rash affecting the vulva and inguinal areas. She has recently completed a course of antibiotics. Her periods are regular, and she has normal bowel and bladder function. She reports a white vaginal discharge.

Diagnostic approach

It is important to note the acute nature of the condition, coexisting medical history and antibiotic use. This makes it likely that the cause is infective or inflammatory.

Examination and Investigations

On examination she has an erythematous eruption affecting the vulva, and there are small white pustules at the periphery of the rash with satellite lesions near the edge. There is a heavy white vaginal discharge. A vaginal swab shows a very high growth of *Candida albicans*.

Diagnostic approach

The heavy discharge suggests an infective cause. Satellite white pustules at the edge of the eruption suggest candida infection. It is important to note that the discharge would be acidic and this can also cause an irritant dermatitis.

Management

Management can be with:
- topical antifungal: clotrimazole pessary or cream
- oral antifungal: severe or recurrent disease
- lifestyle changes: avoidance of soap, use of cotton underwear, salt baths

12.2 Eczema ('dermatitis')

Eczema (also known as dermatitis) may affect the genital area. As discussed in Chapter 9 there are different subtypes of eczema, all of which may present similarly and coexist in the genital area.

Clinical features

Patients present with symptoms of pruritus and dyspareunia together with signs of ill-defined erythema, excoriations and lichenification (**Figure 12.2**). There may be signs of dermatitis elsewhere or a history to suggest a contact source. Some important triggers of genital irritant or contact eczema are listed in **Table 12.1**.

Treatment

Chapter 9 has an extensive discussion of the treatment of eczema. Patients with genital eczema should use emollients regularly at least twice daily, and have a soap substitute prescribed. If there is marked inflammation a low-potency topical steroid should be prescribed for 7–10 days. If there is any evidence of fungal or bacterial infection, this should also be treated with topical agents. Regular antihistamine use may be useful to reduce pruritus.

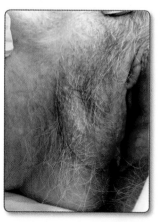

Figure 12.2 Vulval eczema.

Common contact irritants	Common contact allergens
Urine	Topical antibiotics
Faeces	Latex
Hygiene pads	Propylene glycol
Toilet paper dyes	Lidocaine
Detergents	Fragrances

Table 12.1 Common causes of irritant and allergic contact dermatitis

12.3 Psoriasis

Genital psoriasis is the most common male genital dermatosis. It also affects women, but less commonly most patients will have psoriasis affecting other sites, particularly the ear canal, scalp, and elbow and knees; only 3–5% will not have disease elsewhere.

Clinical features

Patients present with well-defined plaques of psoriasis in the genital area and intergluteal cleft. There is usually minimal scaling due to the moist environment (**Figure 12.3**).

Treatment

Patients should use emollients twice daily along with a soap substitute. Topical steroids of mild-to-moderate potency should be used. Topical calcineurin inhibitors may be used instead of steroids topically. In severe cases of isolated genital psoriasis, systemic treatment can be given.

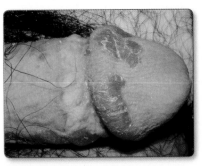

Figure 12.3 Penile psoriasis

12.4 Lichen sclerosus

This is an idiopathic disorder affecting men and women. It is the most common vulval dermatosis and presents in childhood and after age 40 years. There is an association with autoimmune disease, e.g. vitiligo. Both sexes present with pruritus, pain or dyspareunia. Men who develop lichen sclerosus are not usually circumcised. Women with it are at an increased risk of developing vulval squamous cell carcinoma.

Clinical features

Classically there is atrophic hypopigmentation in a 'figure of eight' around the vulva and anal region. There can be purpura, telangiectasia, and loss of normal architecture and hyperpigmentation (**Figure 12.4**). Scarring can occur with narrowing of the introitus and loss of the labia. The loss of anatomical landmarks can make examination difficult.

In men the foreskin and glans are affected, leading to scarring and phimosis. Often minor rubbing or sex can lead to bleeding as a result of skin fragility.

Investigation

Skin biopsy Histology shows a lichenoid inflammatory pattern in early stage lesions or a superficial sclerosing process in late-stage lesions.

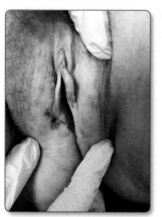

Figure 12.4 Vulval lichen sclerosus.

Treatment

Patients diagnosed with lichen sclerosus should use emollients at least once a day and apply superpotent corticosteroids when disease is active. Women should have annual surveillance for genital squamous cell carcinoma (1–5% lifetime risk). Men are generally treated with circumcision and the lichen sclerosus does not recur.

12.5 Lichen planus

This is an inflammatory condition that can affect the skin, oral and genital mucosa. Vulval lesions are present in half of all women who present with cutaneous lichen planus. The aetiology of lichen planus is unknown. Of patients with severe disease 3% will develop squamous call carcinoma, so routine monitoring is important.

Clinical features

Initial lesions can be painless white patches on the vulva and vagina, and may progress to violaceous, pruritic, painful ulcers that heal with scarring (**Figure 12.5**). In women scarring may lead to narrowing of the introitus and dyspareunia. In severe

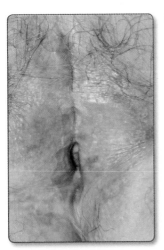

Figure 12.5 Vulval lichen planus.

cases it may preclude cervical smear tests. Lichen planus affects the glans of the penis in men.

There are usually lesions elsewhere so the mouth, scalp, nails and eyes (lacrimal duct) should be examined for lesions and scarring.

Investigation
Skin biopsy Histology shows lichenoid infiltration, hyperkeratosis and pigmentation.

Treatment
Patients should use emollient once daily and have a soap substitute prescribed. In erosive disease, once-daily superpotent topical steroids are often required. In severe disease systemic immunosuppression may be given. Rarely, surgery is required to treat areas of scarring.

> ### Clinical insight
> Severe vaginal scarring due to lichen planus and sclerosus may lead to vaginal stenosis and prevent cervical smear testing. In such cases, vaginal dilators and/or surgery may be required to correct the stenosis.

12.6 Zoon's balanitis

This is a chronic, rare, inflammatory disorder typically affecting middle-aged and elderly men who have not been circumcised. It is frequently associated with lichen sclerosus and patients should be examined carefully for evidence of this.

Clinical features
This condition is relatively asymptomatic. Patients present with sharply demarcated orange–red shiny plaques with 'cayenne pepper' appearance in a 'kissing' distribution.

Investigation
Other causes of irritant balanitis and concomitant lichen sclerosus should be excluded.

Treatment
A mild-potency steroid used once daily for 3 months may help to control disease. Circumcision is a curative treatment.

12.7 Vulvodynia

This is persistent pain of the vulva. Causes such as infection, lichen sclerosus and planus, and neoplasia should always be excluded. Localised vulvodynia causes pain and tenderness at the posterior introitus. Regular use of emollients avoidance of irritants (e.g. wipes, deodorants) and topical anaesthetics may help. In generalised vulvodynia, there is diffuse burning pain with no skin signs. Treatment is as per localised vulvodynia with referral to pain specialists.

12.8 Infections

Yeast and fungal infections

Intertriginous areas provide the optimum environment for these infections. *Candida albicans* is common and presents with white discharge or erythematous pruritic patches with white satellite lesions. Confirmation is with a swab for microscopy and culture, with treatment using either topical or oral antifungals. Differential diagnosis includes erythrasma (*Corynebacterium minutissimum*), which presents with erythematous patches and fine scale.

Sexually transmitted infections

Gonorrhoea is caused by the bacterium *Neisseria gonorrhoeae*; typical symptoms include a purulent green discharge and dysuria. Complications include pelvic inflammatory disease, arthritis, ophthalmia neonatorum and perihepatitis. Treatment is with antibiotics, e.g. ceftriaxone.

Syphilis is caused by the spirochaete *Treponema pallidum*. If untreated it progresses through four stages. Primary syphilis occurs about 3 weeks after inoculation, with a painless chancre and lymphadenopathy. Secondary syphilis presents a few months later with flu-like symptoms and a non-pruritic, widespread, papulosquamous eruption involving the palms and soles (**Figure 12.6**). Alternative presentations include annular plaques, moth-eaten alopecia and crusted necrotic lesions. Mucosal ulcers may also be present with genital condylomata lata. Investigation is with dark-field microscopy

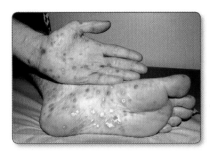

Figure 12.6 Secondary syphilis.

and testing for treponemal antibodies. Treatment is with benzylpenicillin.

Infestations

Crab lice (*Pthirus pubis*) or scabies (*Sarcoptes scabiei*) can occur on the genitals and both present with marked pruritus. Lice can also be seen on the eyelashes at the base of hairs. Scabies gives erythematous papules and nodules (**Figure 12.7**), burrows and crusting, also affecting axillae, finger and toe web spaces. Scraping demonstrates mites, eggs or faecal matter. Treatment of both is with either two applications of topical agents, e.g. permethrin, 1 week apart or oral ivermectin. It is essential to treat all people with close contact to avoid reinfection.

Viral infections

Herpes simplex virus (HSV), usually HSV-2, is a common infection presenting with recurrent painful grouped vesicles on an

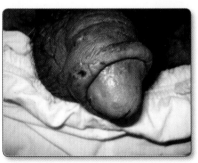

Figure 12.7 Penile scabies.

erythematous base; these subsequently ulcerate. In primary infection there are extensive bilateral crops of blisters in the genital area, with tender lymphadenopathy and a flu-like prodrome. Investigation is with a viral swab. Treatment is with antiviral agents, e.g. aciclovir. Human papillomavirus (HPV) is another common infection (**Figure 12.8**) that causes condylomata acuminata, appearing similar to condylomata lata or molluscum contagiosum. Treatments include podophyllotoxin, imiquimod, cryotherapy or surgery.

12.9 Benign lesions

The following are common benign lesions affecting genital skin:

- Peyronie's disease is a scarring penile disorder of the sheath of tissue surrounding the corpora cavernosa. It affects up to 5% of men. Scarring results in excessive bending or curvature of the penis, which interferes with intercourse. Oral agents and surgery can be tried as treatment.
- Pearly papules of the penis are benign papules around the corona of the glans of the penis. No treatment is required, although CO_2 laser or surgical intervention may help, if desired, for aesthetic reasons.

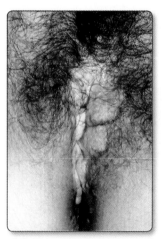

Figure 12.8 Vulval warts caused by the human papillomavirus.

- Epidermoid cysts are frequently found on the labia majora and scrotum. They may be single or multiple; they can be excised if required.
- Bartholin's cysts are found medial to the labia minora, and are commonly caused by blockage of the duct.
- Angiokeratomas (AGKs) can occur in the genital region, as a solitary incidental AGK, part of AGKs of Fordyce or part of Fabry's disease. Solitary lesions can occur in adults, whereas genital lesions occur in both sexes after age 50 years; however, if present in men there may be an underlying urological problem. No treatment is required, but further investigation for male anatomical abnormalities or Fabry's disease should be considered, depending on the distribution of the AGKs, and age and sex of the patient.

12.10 Malignant lesions

Malignant disease may be confined to the epidermis (in situ) or invade the dermis.

In situ disease

The following are examples of in situ disease:
- Vulval/penile intraepithelial neoplasia can be considered with lesions on the genitalia, particularly in patients with a past history of lichen sclerosus, lichen planus or HPV. There may be pruritus, pain or dyspareunia. Given the range of presentations, treatment failure for a presumed benign lesion or a lesion that is growing (**Figure 12.9**) indicates the need for a biopsy. Excision, circumcision or imiquimod may be helpful.

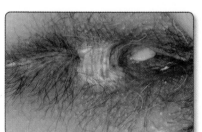

Figure 12.9 Probable in situ malignancy.

- Bowenoid papulosis is a variant of intraepithelial neoplasia, and presents as red–brown papules on the genitalia and thighs.
- Extramammary Paget's disease is a rare intraepithelial adenocarcinoma. It presents with burning or pain in the vulva in women or, in men, in the perianal region; it is associated with a well-defined erythematous plaque that gradually extends. Investigations should include screening for an underlying primary adenocarcinoma elsewhere.

Invasive disease

The following are examples of invasive disease.

- Squamous cell carcinoma can present, in both sexes, with ulcers that have a heaped-up edge; these are non-healing and on the vulva there can be fissuring, nodules or plaques.
- Melanoma is the second most common neoplasia, although about 25% can be amelanotic and so could mimic non-pigmented nodules such as haemorrhoids
- Genital basal cell carcinomas are rare, although they do occur. Investigation is by biopsy of suspicious lesions and treatment is with surgery (Mohs' micrographic surgery), radiotherapy or topical immunotherapy, depending on the histological diagnosis and circumstances of the patient

Hair and nails

The average human scalp contains about 150,000 hairs which are made of keratin and grow in a cyclical fashion divided into four stages (**Table 13.1**). Hair grows at a rate of around 0.4 mm/day.

Understandably patients find hair loss very distressing. Hair loss (alopecia) can be divided into scarring, which is irreversible, and non-scarring forms (**Figure 13.1**). If it is not possible to decide clinically which form of alopecia is present, a scalp biopsy should be performed.

Nails are formed from modified keratin and provide protection to the tips of digits. Fingernails take 6 months to grow from base to tip whereas toenails take 12–18 months. Nail changes may reflect disease confined to the nail, skin disease and/or systemic disease.

Patients presenting with symptoms confined to the hair or nails should always have a full skin examination to seek out clues or signs of disease elsewhere.

13.1 Clinical scenario

A 52-year-old woman presents with an 8-month history of scalp itch and hair thinning. Her hairdresser has commented that her scalp is red.

Stage	Length of stage	Approximate percentage of follicles in stage
Anagen: 'growth phase'	7 years	>80
Telogen: 'resting phase'	3 months	14
Catagen: 'degenerative phase'	2 weeks	2
Exogen: 'shedding phase': occurs during telogen-to-anagen transition		

Table 13.1 Hair follicle cycle

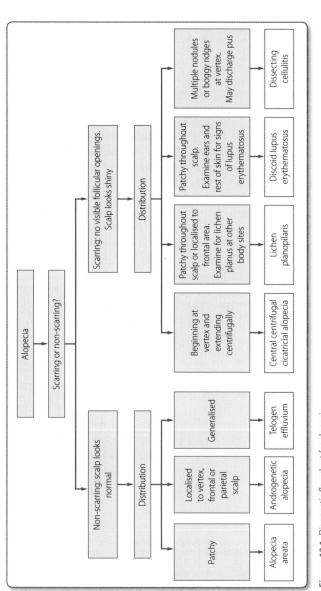

Figure 13.1 Diagnostic flowchart for alopecia.

There are several scattered areas of hair thinning on the scalp. There is loss of follicular openings (scarring), with the remaining hair follicles red and scaly at their opening. On full skin examination there is lateral thinning of three fingernails, with linear ridging but no rash elsewhere, including the mucous membranes.

Diagnostic approach

The history of itch, patchy alopecia, erythema and perifollicular scale suggests an inflammatory scalp disorder leading to follicular destruction. The presentation and the associated nail changes suggest lichen planopilaris.

Investigation and treatment

Given the scale and erythema, fungal infection must be excluded (see page 167). A biopsy of the scalp reveals a lichenoid infiltration and a diagnosis of lichen planopilaris is made. Initially the patient is given superpotent topical steroid scalp lotion. If this fails to control the disease, oral corticosteroids could be given as a short course. For refractory disease a steroid-sparing agent such as ciclosporin could be considered.

13.2 Non-scarring alopecia

Alopecia areata

This is an autoimmune disease characterised by patchy non-scarring alopecia, which is extremely distressing for patients. The lifetime risk of developing alopecia areata is 1–2%. One in five patients has a family member with the same condition. Differential diagnoses include tinea capitis (see page 168) and trichotillomania.

Clinical features

Patients present with abrupt onset of asymptomatic, patchy, non-scarring hair loss from any body site, most commonly the scalp (**Figure 13.2**). Broken 'exclamation-mark' hairs with tapered proximal end are often seen. Nail pitting may be present. Alopecia totalis is loss of all hair from the scalp; alopecia universalis is loss of all hair from the body.

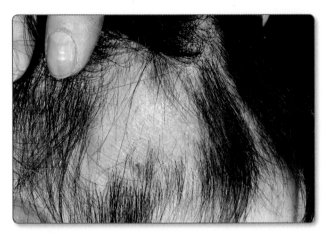

Figure 13.2 Alopecia areata.

Treatment

Limited disease (<50%)

For this:

- no treatment may be necessary
- superpotent topical steroid applied to the area of hair loss may be used
- intralesional steroid injections can be used but the patient should be counselled on the side effects of atrophy and depigmentation

Extensive disease (>50%)

For this, use:

- short courses of an oral steroid
- topical immunotherapy, e.g. diphencyprone
- systemic immunosuppressants, e.g. ciclosporin, methotrexate
- photochemotherapy
- a wig

Telogen effluvium

Events such as pregnancy, severe physical or psychological stress, or chemotherapy may cause most follicles to enter telogen phase simultaneously, leading to sudden shedding of hair – 'telogen effluvium'. The stress trigger for the event usually occurs 2–4 months before the shedding.

Clinical features

Patients present with sudden-onset, widespread, uniform, scalp hair thinning. Hair loss is asymptomatic and the scalp appears normal.

Treatment

With removal of the precipitant, complete regrowth is expected.

Androgenetic alopecia

This hereditary trait is visible in 80% of men by the age of 70 years, although it can affect women too. It is mediated by dihydrotestosterone activity. Early or severe disease should prompt investigation for pathological hyperandrogenism: polycystic ovary syndrome and androgen-secreting tumours of the ovary or adrenal gland.

Clinical features

Male pattern hair loss is characterised by symmetrical, progressive, non-scarring alopecia affecting the frontoparietal and/or vertex region.

Female pattern hair loss may occasionally follow the same pattern but more commonly there is diffuse central thinning of the crown, with preservation of the surrounding hairline.

> **Clinical insight**
>
> Biochemical tests for hyperandrogenism are serum androgens and 17-hydroxyprogesterone. Pelvic ultrasonography and adrenal imaging may be required depending on the results.

Treatment

Options include:
- topical minoxidil 2% or 5% in the first instance
- oral finasteride for men and women with hyperandrogenism
- oral spironolactone for women with hyperandrogenism
- oral contraceptive pill for women with hyperandrogenism

13.3 Scarring alopecia

Central centrifugal cicatricial alopecia

This is characterised by a slowly progressive scarring alopecia, starting at the vertex. It is almost exclusive to patients of African–Caribbean descent, with a female:male ratio of 3:1.

Virtually all patients have used heat or chemical-based styling practices before disease onset, although progression of the disorder is not stopped by avoidance of these techniques.

Clinical features

The alopecia starts at the vertex and extends in a centrifugal pattern (**Figure 13.3**). It is usually asymptomatic but patients may experience mild itch or tenderness. Occasionally pustules may be seen. Longstanding disease may lead to scarring alopecia.

Treatment

A combination of long-acting oral tetracycline antibiotic with a potent topical steroid is most commonly used.

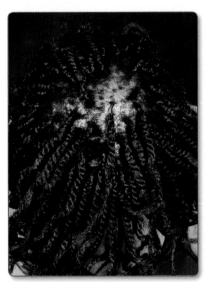

Figure 13.3 Central centrifugal cicatricial alopecia.

Lichen planopilaris

This variant of lichen planus presents as an inflammatory scarring alopecia. It is most common in white women. The main differential diagnosis is discoid lupus erythematosus.

Clinical features

Patients develop itchy patches of scarring alopecia. There is erythema of the involved scalp and perifollicular scale. Lichen planus is found at other body sites in <30% of patients. All patients should be examined for the presence of mucosal and nail lichen planus.

Frontal fibrosing alopecia is the development of lichen planopilaris on the frontal scalp and eyebrows.

Treatment

Initial treatment Superpotent topical steroid is first line; with aggressive disease oral steroids can be initiated.

Severe or refractory disease Either hydroxychloroquine is initiated or immunosuppressive steroid-sparing agents (ciclosporin, azathioprine and mycophenolate mofetil).

Discoid lupus erythematosus

Lesions commonly occur on the scalp, face, ears and neck. Only a small minority of these patients will ever develop systemic lupus. The main differential is lichen planopilaris.

Clinical features

Discoid lupus presents with painful or itchy annular alopecia. Lesions are erythematous and scaly, with dyspigmentation and evidence of follicular plugging (**Figure 13.4**). The patient should be examined for discoid lesions at other sites, and serology to exclude systemic lupus erythematosus (SLE) should be conducted.

Treatment

Treatment may be topical or systemic, based on disease severity. Superpotent topical steroids can be used initially, and hydroxychloroquine is used first line.

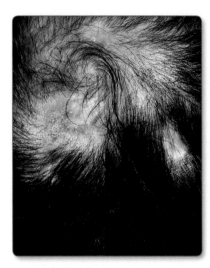

Figure 13.4 Discoid lupus erythematosus.

Dissecting cellulitis of the scalp

This is most common in young African–Caribbean men; it may occur in isolation or with conditions such as acne conglobata, hidradenitis suppurativa and pilonoidal sinus.

Clinical features

Multiple nodules appear on the posterior and vertex of the scalp and rapidly coalesce to form boggy ridges. Foul-smelling pustular discharge is characteristic. Although the appearance suggests infection, the condition is sterile and any cultured bacteria are likely to reflect secondary colonisation.

Treatment

All patients should use a chlorhexidine wash to decrease skin colonisation. Tetracycline antibiotics are used for 3- to 6-month periods. Isotretinoin is useful in the long term. Surgical intervention may be required for deep-seated cystic formation.

13.4 Hirsutism

This is excessive growth of terminal hairs in a male pattern occurring in a woman as a result of hyperandrogenism or increased end-organ androgen sensitivity. It affects 5% of women of reproductive age.

Clinical features

Female patients develop hair growth in a male pattern including the beard area and anterior chest.

Investigations

Underlying causes of hirsutism must be excluded: thyroid function tests (thyroid disease), prolactin level (hyperprolactinaemia), blood glucose (insulin resistance), androgen profile (PCOS) and, if appropriate, dexamethasone suppression test for Cushing's syndrome.

Treatment

Physical treatments, e.g. epilation, shaving, waxing and laser hair removal, are the mainstay of treatment.

> **Clinical insight**
>
> Hirsutism is the abnormal growth of excess terminal hairs in a male pattern in a female patient.
>
> Hypertrichosis is excessive growth of hair in a normal distribution.

If underlying causes are found these should be treated as follows.

- Spironolactone and cyproterone acetate may be used for hyperandrogenism
- Finasteride is used to inhibit 5α-reductase.
- Metformin if hirsutism is associated with insulin resistance.

13.5 Nail disease

Nail abnormalities may occur because of primary nail disorders or infections, be part of a generalised skin disorder or reflect systemic disease.

Nail signs in intrinsic nail disease, cutaneous disease and systemic disease are summarised in **Tables 13.2–13.4**. Treatment for these conditions is generally for the underlying causes.

Sign	Appearance	Cause
Green nails	Green discoloration of one or more nails	Pseudomonas or *Candida* infection
White patches	Distal lateral part of some nails are white with onycholysis, thickening and subungal debris	Dermatophyte or yeast infection
Black or brown patches	Area under nail appears black or brown	Haemorrhage, naevus, melanoma – look for Hutchinson's sign; pigmentation of adjacent cuticle in melanoma

Table 13.2 Nail signs in intrinsic nail disease

Sign	Appearance	Cause
Pitting	Small depressions in nails	Psoriasis – salmon patches and onycholysis (lifting of nail from nailbed) may also be seen; eczema, alopecia areata
Ridging	Longitudinal ridges in nails. Other associated changes: thinning, distal splitting, subungal hyperkeratosis	Lichen planus

Table 13.3 Nail signs in cutaneous disease

Sign	Appearance	Cause
Clubbing	Loss of angle between proximal nail and adjacent skin	Lung malignancy, chronic suppurative lung disease, cyanotic heart disease, malabsorption including inflammatory bowel disease, thyroid disease, pregnancy
Ragged cuticles	Loss of normal smooth cuticle appearance. Visible telangiectasia	Autoimmune connective tissue disease, e.g. systemic lupus erythematosus, dermatomyositis, mixed connective tissue disease, systemic sclerosis
Beau's lines	Transverse grooves	Major physical or psychological stress Chemotherapy
Koilonychia	Spoon-shaped nail	Iron deficiency
Mees' lines	Transverse white lines	Arsenic poisoning
Lindsey's nail (half-and-half nail)	Proximal nail white; distal nail pink/brown	Chronic renal failure
Splinter haemorrhage	Small linear red marks under nail	Infective endocarditis
Yellow nails	All 20 nails appear yellow and thickened	Yellow nail syndrome – associated with bronchiectasis and lymphoedema

Table 13.4 Nail signs in systemic disease

Paediatric dermatology

This broad subspecialty encompasses infectious, atopic and genetic diseases. It is the basis of a high percentage of consultations for GPs and paediatricians. Many of the diseases that occur in children are covered not only in this chapter but throughout the book.

14.1 Clinical scenario

Rash

Presentation

A 4-year-old boy presents with a 24-hour history of rash and fever. He has been unwell for 3 days with fever, coryzal symptoms and anorexia. The rash started on his face and has spread to involve his trunk, arms and thighs.

Diagnostic approach

The history of rash and fever in a child strongly suggests an infectious process, most probably viral.

Examination and investigations

On examination he is unwell with a fever of 39°C and a widespread morbilliform, blanching rash with sparing of the palms and soles (**Figure 14.1**). He has inflamed conjunctivae, pharynx and oral mucosa. There are whitish elevations on the buccal mucosa and generalised lymphadenopathy.

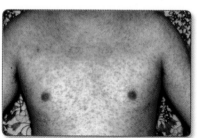

Figure 14.1 Morbilliform rash.

An infectious screen should be sent including serology for atypical pneumonia, rubella and parvovirus B19. Viral swabs should be taken from the buccal mucosa and sent to the lab for polymerase chain reaction (PCR) analysis.

Diagnostic approach

These features are suggestive of measles infection but the differential diagnosis is wide (**Table 14.1**). Typically patients have a prodromal illness for 2–8 days with coryzal symptoms or upper respiratory tract infection and fever. Key features are the morbilliform rash with cephalocaudal spread and sparing of palms and soles, conjunctivitis and changes on the buccal mucosa (Koplik's spots).

> **Clinical insight**
>
> Immunisation remains the safest and most effective method of preventing measles.

It is important to perform a full septic screen and take a thorough drug history. Bloods may show a leukopenia and a thrombocytopenia. Serious complications include pneumonitis and encephalitis.

14.2 Neonatal disease

Erythema toxicum neonatorum

This is a benign vesiculopustular disorder that occurs in full-term infants; it is thought to be secondary to immaturity of the pilosebaceous unit. It is estimated to occur in between 40 and 70% of infants.

Type	Causes
Viral infection	Rubella, Epstein–Barr virus, parvovirus B19, human herpesvirus-6, HIV-1, measles
Bacterial infection	*Mycoplasma pneumoniae*, group A *Streptococci*
Other	Drug reaction, autoimmune connective tissue disease

Table 14.1 Differential diagnosis of morbilliform rash

Clinical features

Patients present with multiple erythematous macules and papules which rapidly form pustules (**Figure 14.2**), mainly on the trunk and limbs, but spare the palms and soles. These occur within 48 hours of birth and resolve within 5–7 days.

Treatment

This condition resolves spontaneously and no specific treatment is required. Culture of pustules for bacterial, fungal and viral causes can be obtained if necessary.

Milia

These are white papules on the skin, frequently on the nose and cheeks (**Figure 14.3**). They are thought to occur due to retention of keratin in the pilosebaceous unit. They resolve within the first few weeks of life.

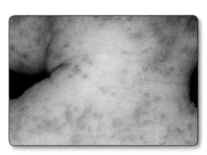

Figure 14.2 Erythema toxicum neonatorum.

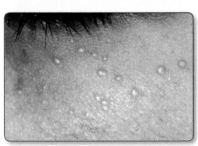

Figure 14.3 Milia.

Transient neonatal pustulosis

This is a benign vesicopustular disorder. It usually affects infants with type VI skin.

Clinical features

Patients present with non-inflammatory pustules that are present from birth; when these rupture, there are erythematous macules with a surrounding collarette of scale. There is residual hyperpigmentation which may take months to resolve.

Treatment

No specific treatment is required and parents can be reassured.

14.3 Infant dermatosis

Seborrhoeic dermatitis

This is a self-limiting rash that occurs in infants from age 3 weeks and is most common around age 3 months. It affects areas with high concentrations of sebaceous glands, e.g. centre of face, external ear, axillae and inguinal folds. Differential diagnoses are atopic dermatitis, psoriasis, napkin dermatitis and tinea capitis.

Clinical features

Infants are well with a normal appetite. The sites specifically affected are:

- **'cradle cap':** greasy, non-inflammatory yellow scales on the scalp
- **facial involvement:** erythematous papules and plaques on the forehead, eyebrows, cheeks and nasolabial folds
- **intertriginous involvement:** confluent shiny erythema in the axillae, neck, inguinal folds and buttocks

Treatment

Parents should be reassured that this is a common, harmless, self-limiting condition.

For 'cradle cap' use emollients to remove scales and ketoconazole 2% shampoo twice weekly. Agents such as hydrocortisone 1%/miconazole 2% may be used twice daily for a week in difficult cases.

For body sites, use of ketoconazole cream 2% or low-potency topical steroid (hydrocortisone 1%/miconazole 2%) and liberal emollients for a week should clear the eruption.

Atopic dermatitis (atopic eczema)

This is common in childhood and estimated to affect up to 20% of children worldwide. The incidence is higher in urban areas and western societies. In 40% of cases it clears by adulthood. Differential diagnoses include scabies infection, seborrhoeic dermatitis, drug reactions and an allergic contact dermatitis.

Clinical features

Patients have dry skin, with itchy, red, scaly lesions on the flexural surfaces and prominent involvement of the antecubital and popliteal fossae. In infants the eczematous rash can involve the extensor surfaces, cheeks and forehead. Lesions may become golden and crusted, usually indicating infection (impetiginisation, often secondary to infection with *Staphylococcus aureus*). The skin may become lichenified as a result of the chronic itch.

Patients should have viral and bacterial swabs performed and skin scrapings taken to exclude scabies infection.

Treatment

In all cases there should be regular use of emollients with topical steroid use on inflammatory lesions (see page 128). Topical calcineurin inhibitors can be used as maintenance treatment. An antibacterial wash and oral antibiotics can be used in cases of infection

> ## Clinical insight
>
> Eczema herpeticum presents with punched-out erosions with crusting and vesicles (see page 144). Prompt treatment with an antiviral agent is essential.

In severe, refractory cases, phototherapy or systemic treatment with immunosuppressants can be given.

Napkin dermatitis

This term is synonymous with 'nappy rash'. It occurs in up to 35% of children and is most common between the age of 9 and 12 months. Most commonly it is due to an irritant dermatitis

Type	Appearance
Irritant dermatitis	Erythema, papules, superficial erosions on areas of skin in direct contact with the nappy. There is sparing of skinfolds
Candida dermatitis	'Beefy' red plaques, papules and pustules with satellite papules at the edge of the eruption in the skinfolds. Tends to occur when irritant dermatitis present for >3 days
Seborrhoeic dermatitis	Well-circumscribed papules and plaques prominent in inguinal creases. Usually child has cradle cap change and flexural involvement
Bacterial infection	Pustules and golden-crusted papules and erosions in the inguinal creases
Langerhans' cell histiocytosis	Recurrent napkin dermatitis with red/orange scaly papules with erosions. Can resemble seborrhoeic dermatitis. Associated with lymphadenopathy, hepatosplenomegaly and anaemia

Table 14.2 Napkin dermatitis

caused by chronic mechanical irritation from the nappy and a cycle of wetness and dryness.

Causes and clinical features are outlined in **Table 14.2**.

Treatment

For irritant dermatitis thick emollients such as paraffin-based preparations should be used regularly. Low-potency topical steroid/antifungal preparations such as hydrocortisone 1%/miconazole 2% may be used twice daily for 3–5 days in more severe cases.

If candidal infections are suspected, topical antifungal agents such as nystatin, clotrimazole or miconazole must be used until the rash resolves.

Treatments for seborrhoeic dermatitis and atopic dermatitis are discussed on pages 242 and 243.

14.4 Infections

Warts

Cutaneous warts, or verrucae, are the clinical manifestation of infection of keratinocytes by the human papillomavirus (HPV).

They are common in children and predisposing factors include atopic dermatitis and immunosuppression.

Clinical features

Warts can occur anywhere on the body, including the palms and soles. Their morphology is variable and includes flat warts, well-defined keratotic papules and filiform warts. Lesions may be single or within groups. Diagnosis is a clinical one and no specific investigations are required.

Treatment

Sixty per cent of warts undergo spontaneous resolution and care should be taken to avoid scarring in any attempts to remove them. The first-line recommendation is occlusion with duct tape and topical salicylic acid preparations. For resistant lesions use topical imiquimod, liquid nitrogen therapy (cryotherapy), laser therapy or surgery.

Molluscum contagiosum

This cutaneous infection is common in childhood and is estimated to occur in 5% of children in the USA. In adults it is associated with immunosuppression and is regarded as a sexually transmitted infection. Molluscum is caused by a pox virus.

Clinical features

There are flesh-coloured, dome-shaped papules (**Figure 14.4**). These papules are up to 5 mm in diameter and shiny with a central indentation (umbilicated). They occur on the

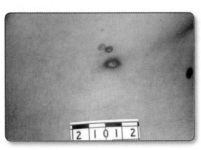

Figure 14.4 Molluscum contagiosum.

trunk and limbs with sparing of the palms, soles and mucous membranes.

Diagnosis is a clinical one and no specific investigations are required.

Treatment

This is a self-limiting disease which usually resolves within 12 months. Aggressive treatment regimens should be avoided to minimise scarring. Topical therapy with 5% potassium hydroxide can be used.

Measles

See Clinical scenario 14.1 (page 239).

Chickenpox (varicella-zoster virus)

This is caused by a double-stranded DNA herpes virus, the varicella-zoster virus (VZV). Infection is spread by droplets via nasopharyngeal secretions. Typically a primary infection occurs in childhood, it is a highly infectious disease and follows a benign, self-limiting course in most cases.

Clinical features

Patients have a prodromal illness of fever, malaise and pharyngitis. Within 24 hours a macular rash appears, which quickly becomes papular and finally vesicular. Crops of vesicles are widespread and classically spread in a cephalocaudal manner. Between 4 and 6 days after onset the vesicles start to crust over.

Patients should be regarded as highly infectious until all lesions have crusted over. Secondary bacterial infection may occur, particularly if the lesions are very pruritic.

Systemic complications are rare but include encephalitis, pneumonia and hepatitis. These more commonly occur in adults with primary VZV infection but may occur in immunocompromised children.

Treatment

Supportive treatments should be instigated with oral fluids and paracetamol. If there is secondary bacterial infection this should be treated. The use of antiviral therapy is not routine in immunocompetent children.

Parvovirus

This is caused by a single-stranded DNA virus, parvovirus B19. More than 70% of adults show immunity to B19. People are most infectious before the appearance of the rash. The route of transmission is thought to be via respiratory secretions.

Clinical features

This is a prodromal illness with coryzal symptoms, fever, headache, nausea and diarrhoea. After 2–5 days an erythematous malar rash occurs – hence the name 'fifth disease'. Children have a 'slapped cheek' appearance. A more generalised rash may develop which may be lace like, morbilliform or vesicular. A 'glove-and-stocking' purpuric rash affecting the hands and feet has also been reported.

Parvovirus infection can cause aplastic anaemia in children with sickle cell disease.

> **Clinical insight**
>
> Parvovirus and chickenpox infection may be lethal to the unborn fetus; infected children should be isolated from pregnant women.

Treatment

There is no specific vaccine or antiviral treatment. In the vast majority of cases this is a benign, self-limiting disease and no specific treatment is required. Children may be given bland emollients to soothe their skin, paracetamol and oral fluids.

14.5 Kawasaki's disease

This is a self-limiting vasculitis that occurs in childhood. Skin disease is polymorphous and clinicians should keep this diagnosis in mind for any child with a prolonged, unexplained fever.

Kawasaki's disease is more common in east Asia or in those of Asian descent.

Clinical features

The patient presents with a persistently high fever (>38.5°C), which usually lasts >5 days, and marked erythema of the lips

Clinical insight

Echocardiography is an essential investigation in all children diagnosed with Kawasaki's disease.

and tongue ('strawberry tongue'). There is a non-purulent conjunctivitis and cervical lymphadenopathy. Up to two-thirds of patients have diarrhoea, vomiting or abdominal pain. There can be serious cardiovascular complications.

Bloods show elevated inflammatory markers, normocytic anaemia, elevated platelets and deranged liver function tests in some cases.

Treatment

Supportive measures with fluids and paracetamol should be given. Aspirin is recommended as therapy in the acute phase of the disease. Options for refractory disease are glucocorticoid therapy and intravenous immunoglobulin (IVIG). All patients should be assessed by a cardiologist.

14.6 Infantile haemangiomas

These are benign vascular tumours that are absent at birth and develop during infancy. Infantile haemangiomas occur in about 5% of white children. They should be distinguished from vascular malformations present from birth, e.g. port wine stain (**Figure 14.5**).

Typically the haemangiomas proliferate for several months before starting to involute. Usually involution starts within a year of the lesion's appearance and it may take many years for the lesions to resolve completely.

Patients with five or more haemangiomas are at risk of having visceral haemangiomas and require ultrasonography of extracutaneous sites. The liver is the most commonly affected site, followed by the gastrointestinal tract and brain.

Clinical features

Different types of haemangioma have different characteristics:
- superficial: bright red papule, nodule or plaque; also known as strawberry or capillary haemangioma
- deep: blue, soft, firm swellings

- segmental: red/violaceous patches and plaques that extend over a territory such as the mandible or maxilla

> **Clinical insight**
>
> Any child with a haemangioma in the beard distribution is at risk of having an airway haemangioma, and should be monitored carefully for signs of respiratory compromise.

Treatment

Most haemangiomas do not require specific intervention. Treatment may be instigated if a haemangioma is:

- ulcerated
- at a site that may impair normal development (e.g. periocular) or feeding
- associated with life-threatening complications, e.g. laryngeal haemangiomas

Oral beta-blockers are the mainstay of treatment for infantile haemangiomas.

Pulsed dye laser may be used for superficial haemangiomas but the risks of a general anaesthetic must be balanced against the benefit of the procedure.

14.7 Genodermatoses

A number of genetic diseases have cutaneous signs (**Table 14.3**). Recognition of these signs is part of a successful diagnosis.

Patients should be seen in a specialist centre at a multidisciplinary clinic.

Disease	Cutaneous features
Neurofibromatosis type I	Axillary freckling, six or more café-au-lait macules, cutaneous neurofibromas
Xeroderma pigmentosum	Some subtypes have sunburn on minimal exposure, widespread freckling at a young age and skin cancers in childhood/adolescence
Epidermolysis bullosa	Blistering and skin erosion on minimal trauma; may heal with severe scarring leading to contractures

Table 14.3 Genodermatoses

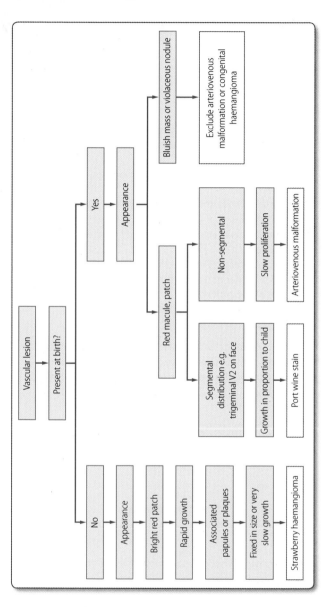

Figure 14.5 Flowchart to distinguish vascular lesions.

Pregnancy-related dermatoses

Skin changes in pregnancy may be physiological, exacerbations of an existing skin condition or a pregnancy-specific dermatosis.

Physiological skin changes are a consequence of hormonal influence and may cause facial hyperpigmentation known as melasma (**Figure 15.1**), striae gravidarum, increased growth of hair and nails, and benign skin tumours (e.g. pyogenic granuloma). Pre-existing skin conditions may become exacerbated or alleviated by pregnancy, e.g. atopic eczema.

Importantly there are some dermatoses that occur only in pregnancy; these are critical to recognise because, rarely, there are associated risks to the unborn child or mother. Most dermatoses of pregnancy resolve postpartum but may occur again in subsequent pregnancies.

When a pregnant woman presents with a dermatosis the following should be established:
- the trimester that symptoms started
- the morphology and distribution of lesions
- a history of skin lesions occurring in previous pregnancies

A skin biopsy and liver function tests are often important to confirm the diagnosis. In some cases the disease may occur in subsequent pregnancies and the woman should be made aware of this.

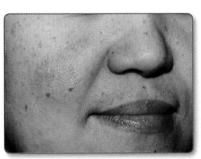

Figure 15.1 Melasma.

15.1 Clinical scenario

Rash in pregnancy

Presentation

A 31-year-old woman, in the early third trimester of pregnancy with her first child, presents with a 1-week history of a pruritic rash that started on her abdomen around her umbilicus and spread quickly to her arms and legs (**Figure 15.2**). She has no previous history of underlying skin disorders.

Diagnostic approach

It is important to note that the patient has no history of an underlying skin disorder that may be exacerbated in pregnancy. She is in her third trimester of pregnancy; this makes a diagnosis of pemphigoid gestationis (PG) or polymorphic eruption of pregnancy (PEP) a possibility. An eruption starting in the periumbilical area is typical of PG.

Examination and investigations

On examination she has urticarial, bullous lesions across the abdomen and limbs. There is no mucosal involvement. A skin biopsy shows a subepidermal blister with eosinophils, and immunofluorescence shows a linear band of complement C3 and immunoglobulin (Ig) G at the basement membrane zone.

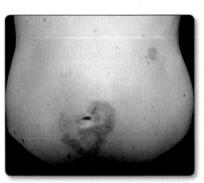

Figure 15.2 Rash in pregnancy.

Diagnostic approach

The key finding of blisters on examination points towards the diagnosis of PG, which is confirmed by the skin biopsy, particularly with immunofluorescence of the pattern seen.

Management

Most patients require a course of oral corticosteroids. Milder disease may be treated with potent topical steroids.

Pemphigoid gestationis has the following complications:

- flare of condition at delivery
- preterm delivery
- 10% risk of neonatal blistering

Clinical insight

One in five cases of pemphigoid gestationis starts postpartum.

15.2 Atopic eruption of pregnancy

This is the most common group of pregnancy-associated dermatoses, occurring in 1 in 150 pregnancies. Atopic eruption of pregnancy (AEP) encompasses a group of atopic disorders that appear or worsen in pregnancy, as a consequence of the immunological changes occurring in the mother during pregnancy to prevent fetal rejection. These changes favour the exacerbation of atopic dermatitis.

The following conditions are types of AEP: atopic dermatitis, prurigo of pregnancy and pruritic folliculitis.

Clinical features

Atopic eruption of pregnancy is more common in first and second trimesters of pregnancy; the skin eruption is eczema like and can affect all parts of the body, including the face, palms, and soles.

Prurigo-like lesions are excoriated papules and nodules on the extensor surfaces of the legs and upper arms. The abdomen can also be involved. There is no risk to the mother or fetus in this condition.

Treatment

Patients should use emollient regularly and may require mild-to-moderate topical steroids regularly for 2–3 weeks. Itchy nodules can be occluded with a dressing to help stop the itch–scratch cycle.

15.3 Polymorphic eruption of pregnancy

This condition occurs in 1 of 160 pregnancies. It was previously known as pruritic urticarial papules and plaques of pregnancy. It is associated with stretching of the skin, often as a result of multiple gestations and high maternal weight gain, usually in the first pregnancy during the third trimester. The stretch of the skin is thought to cause non-antigenic proteins to become antigenic. There is no effect on the fetus.

Clinical features

The eruption starts over the abdomen, commonly involving striae gravidarum with classic sparing of the periumbilical region (**Figure 15.3**). Pruritis coincides with the onset of skin lesions, which are seen as polymorphous, erythematous papules and plaques. The face, palms, soles and mucosal surfaces are usually spared. The lesions resolve in the early postpartum period. The maternal and fetal prognoses are excellent. The diagnosis is a clinical one and investigations are non-specific.

Treatment

Patients should use topical emollients regularly and a moderately potent topical steroid to areas affected by the rash.

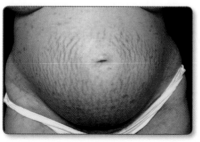

Figure 15.3 Polymorphic eruption of pregnancy.

15.4 Pemphigoid gestationis

This is a rare autoimmune disorder occurring in 1 in 50,000 pregnancies, starting in the second or third trimester. The disease is probably caused by a placental antigen that causes cross-reaction with skin antigens. Complications of preterm labour occur in 20%. The differential diagnoses are bullous pemphigoid, erythema multiforme and PEP.

Clinical features

The skin lesions are intensely pruritic, erythematous, urticarial patches and plaques which progress to form blisters, usually starting in the periumbilical area before the rest of the body becomes affected. Mucosal lesions occur in <20%. Dramatic flares can occur immediately postpartum.

Investigations

The investigations used are:
- skin biopsy – subepidermal blistering
- direct immunofluorescence (DIF) – C3 deposition at the basement membrane zone

Treatment

Most patients require systemic steroids and prednisolone is usually started at a dose of 0.5–1 mg/kg per day. Regular antihistamines may also be used to reduce pruritus. If the disease is very mild, potent topical steroids may be sufficient to control it.

> **Clinical insight**
>
> Pemphigoid gestationis is associated with preterm delivery and neonatal blistering. It is essential to inform the obstetric team of this diagnosis.

15.5 Intrahepatic cholestasis of pregnancy

Intrahepatic cholestasis of pregnancy (ICP) is a reversible, hormonally influenced cholestasis, usually developing in the third trimester. It is the most common pregnancy-related liver disorder, occurring in 1% of pregnancies. Intrauterine fetal death is associated with the condition after 36 weeks' gestation, particularly with high levels of bile acids. Early recognition and timely delivery with induction at 37 weeks are therefore imperative.

Clinical features

There is generalised pruritus, usually starting on the palmar–plantar surfaces, with no other skin manifestations. It most often presents in the late second or early third trimester of pregnancy. The itch is usually worse at night. The skin lesions are secondary excoriations as a consequence of the pruritus. Jaundice may present 1–4 weeks after the pruritus symptoms. Differential diagnoses include acute fatty liver of pregnancy and pregnancy hepatitis.

Investigations

The investigations used are:
- total serum bile acid levels >10 µmol/L
- liver function tests

Treatment

Patients require close monitoring. Bile acid levels must be taken every 2–3 weeks to guide the timing of delivery (usually 37 weeks). In addition coagulation studies and transaminase levels should be monitored. Bile acid binders such as ursodeoxycholic acid, at a daily dose ranging from 600 mg to 2000 mg, may be given.

Psychodermatology

Psychodermatology covers the interaction of mind and body in relation to skin disease. These disorders can be classified as follows:

- **Primary psychiatric disorders:** patients have self-induced cutaneous disease.
- **Secondary psychiatric disorders:** patients develop anxiety and/or depression due to their skin disease.
- **Psychophysiological disorders:** stressful life events can precipitate flares of established disease, e.g. psoriasis and atopic dermatitis.
- **Cutaneous sensory disorders:** in these cases there is no visible skin disease and patients experience purely sensory change.

Clinical insight

A sixth of patients seen in dermatology will require effective management for psychosocial factors for full treatment of the skin disorder. These factors are:

- anxiety
- depression
- delusions
- obsessions and compulsions

16.1 Clinical scenario

Delusional infestation

A 58-year-old woman presents with a 2-year history of an itching sensation over her forearms and abdomen. She believes that a parasite is living 'under her skin' and has brought a glass jar containing a mixture of material that she believes contains one of the parasites (**Figure 16.1**). She has been scratching and picking her skin, causing some ulceration.

Examination and investigations

On examination there is no evidence of true infestation or underlying cause for pruritus. Samples are sent for microbiology and bloods performed to exclude causes of pruritus such as thyroid disease.

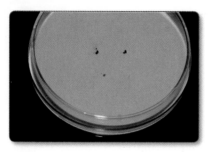

Figures 16.1 Glass box containing 'parasites' from the patient's skin.

Diagnostic approach

It is important to take a full dermatological history and focus on her past medical, travel and psychosocial history. Even though you suspect that the 'parasites' may not be real, they might be! Perform a full dermatological examination, including of the finger webs, and consider a differential diagnosis of a primary skin disorder. The patient should be reassured that you are going to investigate the problem thoroughly.

In this case the appropriate differential diagnoses are:

- true infection or infestation, e.g. scabies
- a primary dermatological condition causing pruritus, e.g. dermatitis herpetiformis
- pruritus secondary to systemic disease, e.g. chronic kidney disease or liver failure
- formication (sensation of crawling on the skin) due to intoxication or drug abuse

The history and clinical features in this case are consistent with a diagnosis of delusional parasitosis. This is a primary psychiatric disorder where a person has a fixed belief that his or her skin is infested with small creatures or parasites. Patients are usually unwilling to see a psychiatrist. Prevalence is estimated at 40/million population, with women more affected than men, and most patients are aged between 50 and 80 years. Individuals give a history of symptoms lasting months or years, usually itching or the sensation of crawling on their skin, which they ascribe to the presence of organisms. They will often treat their skin with disinfectants, and bring samples of skin and other material that they believe represent parasites. Clinical signs range from none at all, to deep excoriations, ulceration and lichenification of multiple areas.

Management

Dermatologists should build a rapport with the patient over several appointments. If the diagnosis is suspected or confirmed it is essential to involve the psychiatry/psychodermatology team. It is advisable not to challenge the patient and discount their beliefs in the dermatology clinic; this should occur in an environment where a psychiatrist is present because they have the appropriate skills and time to explore the origins of the fixed belief, as well as other mental health issues. In some instances an antipsychotic agent such as olanzapine is required to treat the patient's delusion.

16.2 Primary psychiatric disorders

Body dysmorphic disorder

Body dysmorphic disorder (BDD) is a common disorder (up to 1% of the US population) which consists of a distressing preoccupation with an imagined or slight defect in appearance. This can be elicited by asking the patient to draw a self-portrait (**Figure 16.2**). The patient often adopts ritualistic behaviours such as spending excessive amounts of time in front of the mirror to check, hide or improve the perceived physical flaws. This can lead to avoidance of social situations, sexual intimacy and work.

The following differential diagnoses should be considered in cases of BDD:

- anorexia nervosa
- depression
- obsessive–compulsive disorder
- social phobia

Management

The mainstay of therapy is psychotherapy and cognitive–behavioural therapy (CBT). Patients may also take agents such as selective serotonin reuptake inhibitors (SSRIs) or tricyclic antidepressants to aid recovery.

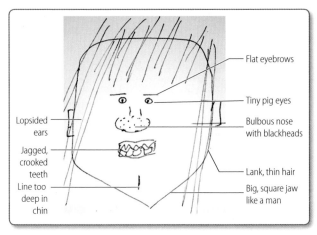

Figure 16.2 Self-portrait of a patient, Anna, aged 19, with body dysmorphic disorder, highlighting multiple perceived flaws.

Dermatitis artefacta

In this condition patients inflict cutaneous lesions upon themselves to satisfy a psychological need, which may be subconscious. When questioned, patients deny any role in the production of the lesions. Dermatitis artefacta (DA) is more common in females, and most cases present in adolescents. The clinical signs are usually accompanied by a fabricated story of how they appeared, making it difficult to diagnose and treat.

Lesions commonly appear on the face, dorsum of the hands and forearm, frequently on the non-dominant limb. Lesions differ depending on the causative agent, e.g. cigarette burns, caustic chemicals, sharp instruments. They may be unilateral or bilateral, and single or multiple (**Figure 16.3**), often in a cluster. There may be scars, vesicles, purpura or ulcers (**Figure 16.4**).

The differential diagnoses in cases of suspected DA include:
• delusional infestation, neurotic excoriations, self-harm

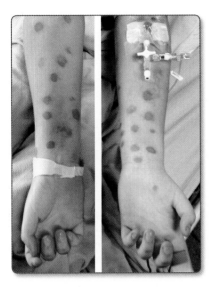

Figure 16.3 Dermatitis artefacta with multiple lesions. This patient has presented with multiple lesions on the forearms.

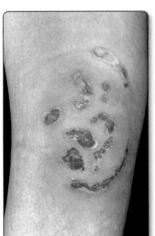

Figure 16.4 Dermatitis artefacta (scars). Note the bizarre-shaped ulcerated lesions. The lesions were caused by the application of a caustic substance with a stick.

- ecthyma
- herpes simplex virus infection
- bullous disorders
- porphyria cutanea tarda
- pyoderma gangrenosum

Management

Optimum management requires input from dermatology specialists and nurses as well as a psychiatric assessment and treatment. The ideal treatment programme includes:

- wound care to assist healing
- exclusion of the possibility of a primary dermatological disorder
- adopting a supportive and non-judgemental approach to treatment
- treating underlying stress and depression
- anxiolytics, antidepressants and low-dose second-generation antipsychotics which may be helpful

Delusional parasitosis

See Clinical scenario 16.1 (page 257).

Nodular prurigo

This is an uncommon, inflammatory dermatosis of unknown aetiology. Patients frequently have a primary psychiatric disorder *and* primary skin disease (atopic eczema). Psychiatric disease such as depression, obsessive–compulsive disorder or emotional distress leads to chronic repetitive scratching or picking of the skin. It mainly affects adults, but occasionally occurs in adolescents and children, especially those with atopic eczema. The differential diagnoses include scabies, recurrent insect bites and lichen planus.

Clinical features

Examination findings consist of multiple, symmetrically distributed, dome-shaped nodules with varying degrees of erosion or ulceration. These are skin coloured but can be darker as a result of post-inflammatory hyperpigmentation (**Figure 16.5**).

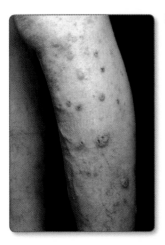

Figure 16.5 Nodular prurigo.

Lesions are typically located on the extensor aspects of the extremities, upper and lower back, and buttocks. The hard-to-reach mid-back is usually spared.

Management
Management includes:
- exclusion of underlying systemic causes of pruritus
- potent topical steroids under occlusion
- phototherapy
- antihistamines to control itch
- treatment directed towards underlying compulsive behaviour

16.3 Secondary psychiatric and psychophysiological disorders

Patients with chronic skin disease, e.g. psoriasis, are thought to be at increased risk of depression, anxiety and suicide because of their skin disease (secondary psychiatric disease).

Chronic skin diseases such as psoriasis may be exacerbated by stressful life events (psychophysiological disorder). There are various factors that can worsen or trigger skin diseases, including emotional stress and alcohol.

Management

Pharmacological interventions in conditions such as psoriasis should be accompanied by:

- regular assessment of dermatology life-of-quality index
- history of alcohol use
- assessment of mood
- patient counselling and education, and involvement of a psychologist to assist with coping mechanisms

Dermatological emergencies

Dermatological emergencies can occur as a primary skin disease or cutaneous manifestations of a systemic disease (discussed in Chapter 11). They can be life threatening and often require intensive supportive care to manage the functions that the failing skin is unable to do. Patients may present dramatically with blistering, skin loss and widespread erythema. Frequently they have tachycardia, hypotension, pyrexia, fluid balance and thermoregulation impairment. In certain cases patients have systemic infection due to the defective skin barrier.

Once the patient is resuscitated it is important to do the following:

- Obtain a full medical and drug history. If the patient cannot give the history, collateral history from a relative or general practitioner should be sought.

> **Clinical insight**
>
> The term 'erythroderma' indicates that >90% of the body surface area (BSA) is red.

- Full skin examination is essential and should include the palms, oral cavity, genitalia, eyes, scalp and soles of the feet.

17.1 Clinical scenario

A 47-year-old man is brought to the accident and emergency department by ambulance with malaise and a rash. His blood pressure is stable, but he is tachycardic with a low-grade fever of 37.8°C. The patient gives a history of worsening rash over the last few weeks. He now has erythema all over his body. He has not taken any new medications or any over-the-counter preparations. Both he and his sister have previously been treated for scalp psoriasis by their GP.

Diagnostic approach

The differential diagnoses for anyone presenting with erythroderma are psoriasis, eczema, drug reaction, pityriasis rubra pilaris and cutaneous T-cell lymphoma (CTCL).

The clues from the history that favour erythrodermic psoriasis are a history of scalp psoriasis and no history of medications.

Examination and investigations

On examination he has erythematous skin on his whole body except his face. There is thick adherent scale on the hands and palms, thickened skin on the body and peripheral oedema. The eyes and mucous membranes are normal. On close inspection of the nails, there is pitting and subungual hyperkeratosis, and the scalp is scaly.

Nail pitting Subungual hyperkeratosis and scale in the scalp are signs of psoriasis.

Investigations required for this patient are:
- to take blood pressure, temperature and pulse regularly
- to monitor fluid balance
- full blood count (FBC), urea and electrolytes (U&Es), liver function tests (LFTs), T-cell count and Sézary's cell count
- swabbing of weeping or open skin
- incisional skin biopsy – haematoxylin and eosin (H&E) stain, immunofluorescence and T-cell rearrangement studies

Clinical insight

Sézary's syndrome is an aggressive variant of CTCL in which malignant leukaemic cells (Sézary's cells) can be detected in peripheral blood.

17.2 Erythroderma

Erythroderma (**Figure 17.1**) refers to redness of the skin involving >90% of its surface. It may be primary, due to a medication or new-onset disease, or secondary, due to a chronic skin condition. It tends to affect men more and occurs in middle age.

Causes of erythroderma (**Figure 17.2**) include:
- psoriasis
- drug reactions
- atopic dermatitis
- pityriasis rubra pilaris
- CTCL/Sézary's syndrome

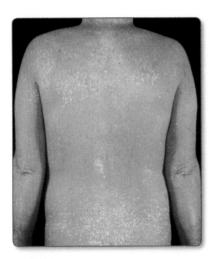

Figure 17.1
Erythroderma.

Clinical features

Patients present with erythema affecting >90% of the body surface area. There is widespread scaling and the skin may be shed in large amounts – exfoliative dermatitis. The patient is systemically unwell with widespread lymphadenopathy, fever and tachycardia.

Investigations

Establishing an accurate diagnosis enables effective treatment of the underlying cause. Investigations to establish the underlying disorder in erythroderma are outlined in Clinical scenario on page 265.

Management

Supportive measures should be instigated immediately and include the following:

- Thick paraffin-based emollients should be applied at 2-hourly intervals to maintain an effective barrier
- The fluid balance should be monitored carefully and insensible losses replaced
- Patients should be nursed carefully with a Bair Hugger

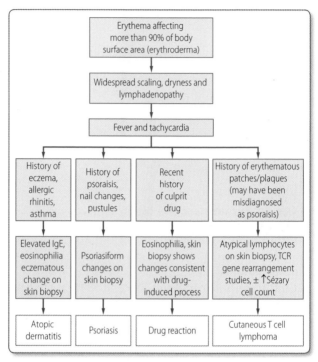

Figure 17.2 Diagnostic flowchart.
Ig, immunoglobulin.

Clinical insight

Pityriasis rubra pilaris is a rare inflammatory condition of the skin characterised by widespread, reddish-orange scaly patches with well-defined borders. The condition may resolve spontaneously.

- Bloods should be taken regularly for electrolytes, FBC and inflammatory markers
- Any infection should be treated with parenteral antibiotics
- Sedating oral antihistamines can be used if the patient is pruritic
  Low-potency topical corticosteroids can be given.

Once the underlying cause of the erythroderma has been discovered, the appropriate systemic therapy should be started.

17.3 Angio-oedema

Angio-oedema is the swelling of the skin and subcutaneous tissues. It can occur with urticaria, anaphylaxis or on its own. Anaphylaxis with angio-oedema of the airway is life threatening and requires the medical emergency team.

Causes of angio-oedema include:

- allergic reactions: immunoglobulin (Ig) E-mediated reactions, e.g. to latex, foods and insect venom
- drugs: non-steroidal anti-inflammatory drugs (NSAIDs), aspirin, opiates, angiotensin-converting enzyme inhibitors, angiotensin II receptor blockers, calcium channel blockers and radiocontrast media
- oestrogens: oral contraceptive pill, hormone replacement therapy and pregnancy
- abnormalities in the level or function of the regulatory C1 esterase inhibitor: these may be congenital or acquired. In the hereditary form there is deficiency of C1 esterase inhibitor from birth. The acquired form presents later in life and is associated with lymphoproliferative disorders

Once immediate life support has been given it is essential to take a careful history of previous episodes, current medications and family history.

Differential diagnoses include cellulitis/erysipelas, facial lymphoedema, autoimmune conditions (systemic lupus erythematosus [SLE], dermatomyositis) and hypothyroidism.

Clinical features

Patients present with widespread, urticarial, erythematous plaques on any body site. These tend to be painful and itchy. There is marked periorbital swelling (**Figure 17.3**) which can preclude eye opening. Gross swelling of the lips may be unilateral (**Figure 17.4**). Tongue and pharyngeal swelling can lead to stridor. Colicky abdominal pain can occur due to swelling of the bowel wall.

> **Clinical insight**
>
> Patients with angio-oedema may rapidly develop airway obstruction due to laryngeal swelling.

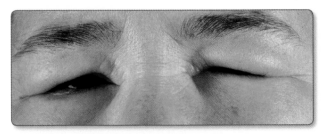

Figure 17.3 Periorbital swelling in angio-oedema.

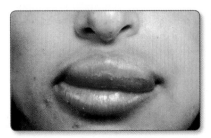

Figure 17.4 Lip swelling in angio-oedema.

Treatment

Assess the patient according to the airway, breathing and circulation (ABC) algorithm. If there is any evidence of airway compromise an anaesthetist must attend immediately.

If anaphylaxis is suspected give 0.5 mg adrenaline (0.5 mL of 1:1000) intramuscularly. Fluid resuscitation is with intravenous fluids and, if there is bronchospasm, bronchodilators should be given. Intramuscular/intravenous chlorphenamine 10 mg and intravenous hydrocortisone 200 mg should be administered and the patient may require monitoring in a high-dependency unit.

The underlying cause of angio-oedema should be identified and appropriate management initiated, e.g. cessation of the causative agent, replacement of C1 esterase inhibitor.

17.4 Blistering eruptions

Blistering disorders can be divided according to the aetiology:
- death of epidermal cells: toxic epidermal necrolysis (TEN) or erythema multiforme

- excessive oedema within the epidermis: acute allergic contact dermatitis (see page 105)
- destruction of adhesion molecules within epidermis: autoimmune blistering disorders such as bullous pemphigoid and pemphigus vulgaris (see page 140)

There are a number of dermatological emergencies that may present with epidermal detachment. Positive Nikolsky's sign is seen in these conditions. With all blistering disorders, swabs of blister fluid should be sent for microbiology and virology, and a skin biopsy with direct immunofluorescence taken. Full investigations should be for the underlying cause of sepsis and any suspected medication should be discontinued.

As with all dermatology cases, a careful drug and medical history will guide your differential diagnosis. Ask about any prodromal symptoms such as an itchy urticarial rash in the preceding weeks, as described in bullous pemphigoid. A drug history for the last 12 weeks is essential.

Treatment

Patients with life-threatening blistering disorders are often systemically unwell and may require care in an HDU. Close monitoring of the blood pressure, fluid balance and temperature, and regular skin inspection are crucial.

> **Clinical insight**
>
> Nikolsky's sign is positive if the epidermis can be detached through the exertion of light tangential pressure on the skin. A blister forms within minutes.

Supportive measures (see section 17.2, page 266) should be given. If there are tense painful blisters, a sterile needle should be used to lance them but leave the blister roof in place.

17.5 Purpura fulminans

This is a rare, rapidly progressive syndrome of intravascular thrombosis and haemorrhagic infarction of the skin. Patients are usually extremely unwell and often require care on an HDU. The condition may occur as a result of trauma, malignancy, sepsis or obstetric complications.

Clinical features

Patients are unwell (tachycardia, hypotension, fever, fluctuating level of consciousness) and present with widespread branching purpura on the skin with areas of associated blistering (**Figure 17.5**). The branched shape reflects the distribution of the vascular network supplying the skin. Purpura in this distribution is called *retiform purpura*. There is disseminated intravascular coagulation (DIC), which is due to abnormal activation of the clotting cascade, leading to consumption of clotting factors. There is extensive thrombosis and haemorrhage.

Investigations

It is essential that a full septic screen be sent along with the FBC, U&Es, LFTs, full clotting profile and vasculitic screen. In neonatal purpura fulminans, a chromogenic assay is necessary to assess the endogenous activity of proteins C and S and antithrombin III.

A skin biopsy is performed in almost all patients to help identify the cause.

Treatment

Supportive measures as outlined in section 17.2 should be instigated. Patients usually require intensive care unit (ICU)/HDU care for fluid monitoring, intravenous antibiotics, inotropes and intensive skin care. In neonatal purpura fulminans,

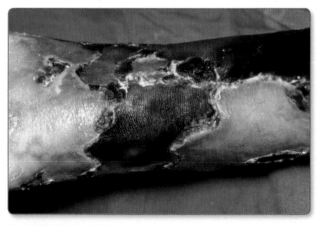

Figure 17.5 Purpura fulminans.

an immediate platelet concentrate should be given. Any dead tissue should be debrided.

Prompt identification of the underlying cause is essential to achieve curative treatment.

17.6 Staphylococcal scalded skin syndrome

Staphylococcal scalded skin (SSS) syndrome is a condition seen in children and infants aged <5 years. Particular strains of *Staphylococcus aureus* release epidermolytic toxins; these break the epidermal cell adhesion molecule desmoglein 1, and lead to superficial skin erosions and blistering. SSS syndrome rarely affects adults, but may be seen in immunocompromised patients.

Clinical features

Patients present with a prodromal pyrexial illness. After this red and tender skin develops, commonly on the face, neck, axillae and perineum. Painful flaccid bullae then develop and rupture easily. Reddened raw-looking skin is present at the blister base; this resembles scalded skin, hence the name of the condition.

In the early stages the differential diagnoses include sunburn and drug reaction. There is an absence of mucosal lesions in SSS syndrome, and swabs are often negative. The skin desquamates and heals without scarring.

Investigations

Swabs should be taken from the blisters for bacteriological confirmation and antibiotic sensitivity. Nasal swabs should be performed of the patient and the family to identify carriers of *S. aureus*.

Treatment

In-patient admission is advised for these cases to offer supportive care to the poorly functioning skin. Analgesia may be required and if paracetamol is not sufficient opioids are preferred to NSAIDs. First-line therapy is anti-staphylococcal antibiotics such as intravenous flucloxacillin.

Monitoring of temperature, fluid balance and urine output is recommended. Blisters should be left intact. Topical therapy is not necessary. Antipyretics should be given as required.

17.7 Eczema herpeticum

This is the rapid dissemination of a herpes simplex virus super-infection over the inflamed skin of patients with pre-existing atopic dermatitis. It is potentially life threatening and most commonly affects children and immunocompromised individuals. The differential diagnosis includes chickenpox.

Clinical features

Patients usually present with fever, malaise and palpable lymphadenopathy. There may or may not be a visible 'cold sore'. There is a vesicular eruption with a predilection for the face and perioral area. The eruption consists of monomorphic punched-out erosions and haemorrhagic crusting (**Figure 17.6**). If the periorbital skin is involved, careful assessment of the eye should be carried out for keratoconjunctivitis and the ophthalmologist should be involved. Lesions heal over a period of 2–6 weeks.

Treatment

Virology and microbiology swabs must be taken from the affected skin. Only bland emollients should be used. Treatment-dose aciclovir should be given five times a day and the course should continue for 14 days. If there is any evidence of bacterial

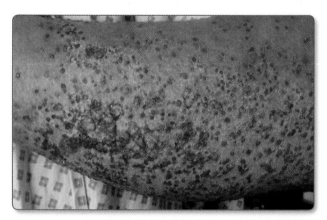

Figure 17.6 Eczema herpeticum.

infection, this should be treated. If the disease is severe medication should be parenteral. Fluid balance should be monitored and analgesia given.

17.8 Stevens–Johnson syndrome and toxic epidermal necrolysis

Stevens–Johnson syndrome and toxic epidermal necrolysis (TEN) are immune complex-mediated hypersensitivity, rare, mucocutaneous syndromes that occur more commonly in patients with HIV and SLE. They are mainly, although not always, caused by drugs. Causes of Stevens–Johnson syndrome/TEN are shown in **Table 17.1**.

There is often overlap between the two conditions, differentiated by the degree of skin and mucosal involvement. Stevens–Johnson syndrome and TEN involve a rash, blistering and mucous membrane involvement (eyes, mouth, genitals) (**Figure 17.7**). The body surface area involved in epidermal detachment ('scalded skin') is the key to differentiating Stevens–Johnson syndrome and TEN (**Figure 17.8**).

Clinical features

There is a prodromal illness of flu-like symptoms for several days before the sudden development of a mucocutaneous, erythematous, painful skin eruption, which starts on the trunk and progresses rapidly. Blisters within the eruption merge and form sheet-like detachment of the epidermis. Nikolsky's sign is positive.

Drugs commonly causing SJS/ TEN	Infections causing SJS/TEN
Allopurinol	Herpes simplex virus
Carbamazepine	Epstein–Barr virus
Sulfonamides	*Mycoplasma pneumoniae*
Abacavir	
Phenytoin	
Non-steroidal anti-inflammatory drugs	

Table 17.1 Causes of Stevens–Johnson syndrome (SJS)/toxic epidermal necrolysis (TEN)

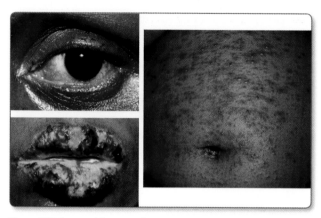

Figure 17.7 Stevens–Johnson syndrome.

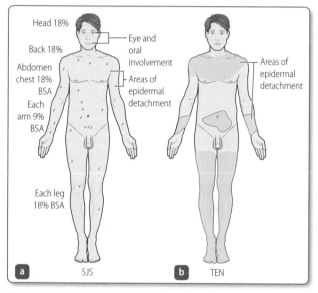

Figure 17.8 Epidermal detachment and body surface area (BSA) in SJS and TEN. (a) If epidermal detachment involves < 10% BSA the patient has SJS. (b) If epidermal detachment involves > 30% the patient has TEN. Between 10–30% BSA epidermal detachment is SJS-TEN overlap syndrome.

The eyes are usually red with photophobia and conjunctivitis. There may be a cough with thick purulent sputum, and dysuria due to genital ulceration.

Investigations

Diagnosis is based on the clinical presentation but can be confirmed on skin biopsy. The skin biopsy will show subepidermal bullae and epidermal necrosis. The following investigations are performed to determine the SCORTEN, which is a severity score to predict the mortality rate. One point is scored for each criterion at presentation. A score of 5 predicts a mortality rate of 90%. The investigations concerned are:

- age >40 years
- presence of a malignancy
- heart rate >120 beats/min
- epidermal detachment >10%
- serum urea >10 mmol/L
- serum glucose >14 mmol/L
- serum bicarbonate <20 mmol/L

Treatment

Potential culprit drugs should be withdrawn immediately. The prognosis in both conditions is proportional to the speed at which the culprit drug is withdrawn. The approach to management is multidisciplinary; there must be involvement of an ophthalmologist, dermatologist, gynaecologist and gastroenterologist to reduce adverse sequelae.

Patients with TEN warrant admission to the ICU for monitoring of fluid balance and infection and support with rigorous skin care (see section 17.2).

Immunomodulation is a controversial area and there is no evidence to suggest that corticosteroids, immunoglobulins and ciclosporin are of any benefit to disease outcome.

Complications

More than half the survivors of TEN will have long-term sequelae, including alopecia, scarring, pigmentary change, nail dystrophy, and vaginal or urethral strictures. Ocular surface sequelae include blindness, photophobia and entropion.

17.9 Necrotising fasciitis

This is a life-threatening infection involving the deep soft tissue of the skin. It is uncommon; risk factors for the disease include trauma to the skin (reduction of skin barrier function) and underlying immunosuppressive diseases. Various bacteria can cause the condition; the important ones to remember are group A streptococci and marine organisms such as *Vibrio* sp. and *Aeromonas hydrophila* (these are particularly virulent and can be fatal within 2 days). The mortality rate is 25%.

Clinical features

Patients are systemically unwell with **severe and constant pain**, usually in a limb; there may be very few skin changes in the early stage. Initially there may be some oedema and erythema, but the severe pain extends beyond these margins (different from cellulitis). Within 2 days the area becomes very firm and the skin discoloured (grey/purple), and haemorrhagic bullae can develop. Crepitus may develop in the affected area. At day 4 there is usually hypotension and septic shock. The main differential diagnosis is cellulitis or pyoderma gangrenosum.

Investigations

The diagnosis is a clinical one with no definitive test. A 'finger test' can be performed – a 2-cm incision down to the fascia is made with insertion and gentle probing by the index finger. In necrotising fasciitis there is malodorous pus, lack of bleeding and little tissue resistance. Cultures should be taken of the pus and the blood. MRI may be useful to show the extent of tissue involvement.

Management

The shocked patient should be resuscitated and urgent surgical debridement of the affected area is required. The debridement must remove ALL infected tissue and therefore is usually extensive. Start high-dose intravenous antibiotics immediately with a regimen to cover streptococci, staphylococci and anaerobes. If *Vibrio* spp. suspected, include tetracycline therapy.

Dermatological surgery

Dermatological surgical techniques play an essential role in the diagnosis and treatment of skin disease. The fundamentals and principles need to be understood for even minor procedures to optimise tissue sampling and cosmetic outcome, and to prevent tumour recurrence.

18.1 Basic concepts in skin surgery

The skin has viscoelastic properties and, if mechanical stress is applied to the skin, mechanical creep (lengthening of the tissue) will occur. The thickness and elasticity of the skin vary depending on the amount of sun exposure that the patient has had, the body site and the patient's age.

Relaxed skin tension lines

Relaxed skin tension lines (RSTLs) of the face and body develop in response to the movement of muscles and other underlying structures (**Figure 18.1**). They correspond to skin wrinkles or crease lines on the face. By closing wounds along or parallel to the RSTLs a narrower and stronger scar results which helps to achieve the best cosmetic result.

RSTLs should not be confused with Langers' lines (mapped in cadavers), dermatomes (spinal nerve innervation) or lines of Blaschko (embryonic development).

> **Clinical insight**
>
> RSTLs are more easily identified by asking the patient to adopt the extremes of facial expression (smiling, squinting or raising the eyebrows).

Cosmetic subunits of the face

During facial surgery one must consider the cosmetic subunits, which correspond to natural junctions between similar areas of skin based on texture, colour, UV exposure, hair and sebaceous content. **Figure 18.2** shows these units. Repairs within one unit or oriented along the natural boundary will produce the best cosmetic results.

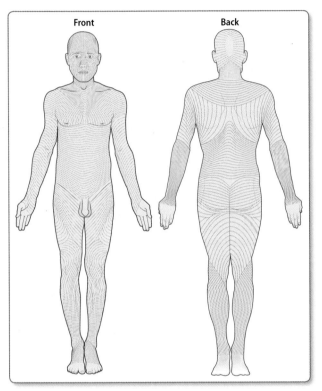

Figure 18.1 Relaxed skin tension lines.

18.2 Anatomy of the soft tissues of the face

Skin layers

The **face** is formed of six layers below the epidermis: dermis, subcutaneous fat, superficial musculoaponeurotic system (SMAS), deep fascia, deep muscles of the face (muscles of mastication) and periosteum. The SMAS is the facial fibromuscular layer that envelopes and interconnects the facial muscles. It

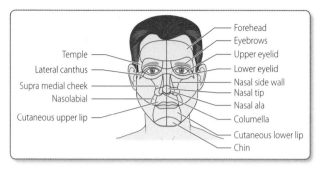

Figure 18.2 Cosmetic subunits of the face.

coordinates facial movements; most of the major vessels and nerves are within or beneath the SMAS. On the face, dissection is usually best performed just above the SMAS.

The **scalp** is formed by memorable layers: skin, connective tissue, galeal aponeurosis, loose areolar tissue, periosteum. Undermining, a technique used to mobilise tissue, should be in the avascular subgaleal zone.

Body sites elsewhere are straightforward, with undermining in the deep fat, just above the fascia.

Nerve supply of the head and neck

Motor supply is via the five branches of the facial nerve. The motor branches are depicted in **Figure 18.3** and the probable sites and consequences of damage in **Table 18.1**. In adults, particular concern is when surgery occurs in the region of:
- the temporal branch of the facial nerve
- the mandibular branch of the facial nerve
- the spinal accessory nerve

Motor nerve damage is rare at other body sites.

Sensory nerves may be divided during surgery; local sensory disturbance often resolves in less than a year. Sensory nerves can also be exploited by nerve blockade for anaesthesia during surgery.

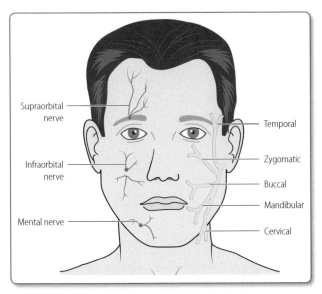

Figure 18.3 Motor and sensory nerve supply of head and neck.

Vascular supply of the head and neck

There are many blood vessels that supply arterial blood (**Figure 18.4**) to and drain venous blood from the head and neck. Extensive anastomoses between vessels in the head and neck mean that there is a negligible risk of ischaemic complications during surgery. Four important vessels may be encountered:

1. superficial temporal artery at the temple (temporal region)
2. facial artery branches (medial canthus and lateral to nasal ala)
3. external jugular vein (over sternocleidomastoid just beneath the platysma)
4. parietal emissary veins (subgaleal space – communicates with intracranial venous sinuses)

Free margins

These are special areas of the face that are discontinuous with adjacent skin. They include the lip, helices, nasal alae, tragus

Structure	Site	Consequence of damage
Temporal branch of facial nerve	From the zygomatic arch as it crosses the temporal region (covered only by fascia)	Inability to elevate eyebrow, ptosis, facial asymmetry
Zygomatic/buccal branches of facial nerve (uncommon)	Medial to anterior border of the parotid along a line drawn from tragus to lateral canthus	Inability to close eye, ectropion/drooling
Marginal mandibular branch of facial nerve	Mandible at the anterior border of the masseter	Unilateral depression of mouth, drooling
Children <5 years Facial nerve – main trunk	Posterior to earlobe – facial nerve lies superficially before the mastoid develops fully	Severe facial paralysis
Spinal accessory nerve	Over sternocleidomastoid at Erb's point (from the midpoint of a line between the angle of the mandible and mastoid process, a vertical line is dropped around 6 cm to the posterior border of sternocleidomastoid)	Shoulder droop, winged scapula, pain
Common peroneal nerve (rare)	Over head of fibula	Foot drop

Table 18.1 Sites and consequences of damages to motor branches of branches of the facial nerve

and eyelid margins. This makes them vulnerable to iatrogenic directional pull. These areas may cause a functional or cosmetic problem if distorted during wound closure.

18.3 Anaesthesia

Local anaesthetics (LAs), classified as amides or esters, are widely used in dermatological surgery. They preferentially block the depolarisation of unmyelinated C (pain) nerve fibres (**Table 18.2**).

Topical anaesthetics

Topical LAs are useful for some procedures and in children before injection of an LA. The most common preparation is

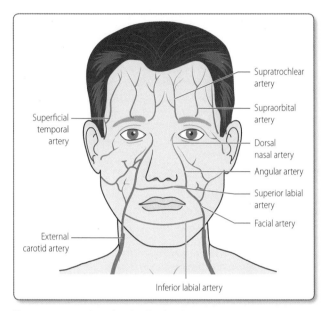

Figure 18.4 Arterial supply to head and neck.

lidocaine 2.5%/prilocaine 2.5% (EMLA – eutectic mixture of local anaesthetics) or tetracaine gel 4% (Ametop), applied under occlusion for >1 h. Tetracaine 0.5% drops can be used for the conjunctiva.

Procedure for LA skin infiltration

Step 1 Perform verbal ('talkaesthesia') and mechanical distraction (squeezing/rubbing the site of injection) and inject warmed solution. Inject slowly using a small syringe (2–5 mL generates less pressure) and a fine-gauge needle (27–30 G).

Step 2 Puncture the skin, aspirating to avoid intravascular injection; inject a small amount as a bleb intradermally (for immediate anaesthesia).

Step 3 Advance the needle through anaesthetised skin, aspirate and inject slowly into the subcutaneous fat. Start proximally and proceed distally.

Local anaesthetic	Proprietary name	Onset (min)	Duration (h)
Amides			
Lidocaine	Xylocaine	Rapid	0.5–2 (4 h with adrenaline)
Bupivocaine	Marcaine	5–8	2-4
Prilocaine (± felypressin)	Citanest (with Octapressin)	5–6	0.5–2
Ropivacaine	Naropin	1–15	2–6
Esters			
Tetracaine	Pontocaine/ Ametop	7	2–3
Procaine	Novocaine	5	1–1.5
NA, not available.			

Table 18.2 Local anaesthetics

Nerve blocks

LA infiltration around sensory nerves may provide additional anaesthesia.

Face Figure 18.3 shows the sites for the following nerve blocks.

- Supraorbital/supratrochlear block: inject 2–5 mL LA superficially and laterally 1 cm medial and just above the supraorbital notch in the midpupillary line.
- Infraorbital block: there are two approaches:
  - cutaneously: injection of 2–5 mL LA perpendicularly into the skin 1 cm inferior to the infraorbital rim in the midpupillary line
  - intraorally (**Figure 18.5**): the upper lip is elevated at the level of the first/second upper bicuspid molars (fourth/ fifth teeth) and 2–5 mL LA injected via a longer (2.5- cm) needle at the site of the infraorbital foramen in the midpupillary line while palpating with the middle finger.
- Mental block: insert the needle into the oral mucosa opposite the second lower bicuspid molar (fifth tooth) in the midpupillary line until bone is reached. Withdraw slightly

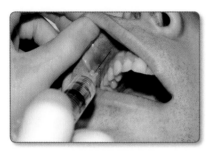

Figure 18.5 Infraorbital nerve block – intraoral approach.

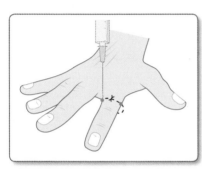

Figure 18.6 Digital nerve block.

and inject 2–5 mL LA.

Ring Digital/ring block: use <3–4 mL plain LA for each digit. The needle is inserted into the digit at a 10 o'clock position and then 2 o'clock on other side (**Figure 18.6**); a bleb is injected at the insertion site, and then advanced along the side of the bone until the needle tip can be palpated from the digital palmar surface; aspirate and then <2 mL is injected into each side, as the needle is withdrawn.

Reactions to LAs may be classed as:

- vasovagal episodes to the procedure
- palpitations secondary to adrenaline
- anaphylactic – to the LA or preservatives
- toxic

LA toxicity

This is more common in children, elderly people and patients with renal/hepatic failure. Symptoms include anxiety, tinnitus, digital tingling, metallic taste, nausea/vomiting, light-headedness, double vision, tremor and convulsions (late). In most cases treatment is supportive ± diazepam. In severe cases (evidence of cardiorespiratory compromise) the arrest team should be called and 20% lipid emulsion may be administered.

18.4 Patient evaluation: informed consent and preoperative assessment

Before surgery the patient should be assessed for suitability and awareness of risks for a given procedure.

Preoperative assessment

At assessment attention should be paid to factors in the patient's history that would mean modifying surgical technique or increasing the risk of complications.

Factors that would a cause modified surgical technique are:
- cardiac disorders (LA)
- pacemaker or implantable defibrillator
- blood-borne infections
- pregnancy – special positioning of patient
Factors that would increase risk of complications are:
- clotting disorders
- diabetes and immunosuppression
- joint replacement due to risk of haematogenous joint infection
- cigarette smoking, which impairs wound healing and increases complications
- history of keloids or hypertrophic scars

Drug history and allergy

It is essential to ask about any history of allergies to medication and dressings to avoid administering culprit allergens to patients.

If a patient is on an anticoagulant agent it is essential to assess the need for this perioperatively. Any anticoagulant agent increases the bleeding during the surgery and postoperatively. The following rules of thumb about anticoagulation may be used:

- warfarin: continue if international normalised ratio (INR) <3
- aspirin/clopidogrel: should be continued; if there is no medical indication for antiplatelets then withhold 10 days before and 5 days after surgery
- non-steroidal anti-inflammatory drugs (NSAIDs): stop if possible (4 days before and 2 days after)
- stop patient taking vitamin E, fish oils, liquorice, gingko biloba, ginger and feverfew

Antibiotics

Routine use of antibiotics after skin surgery is not recommended. Surgery involving the following is the exception:

- breach of oral mucosa
- surgery at an infected site
- if there is a high risk of infection; high-risk areas for infection: below the knee, wedge resection ear/lip, skin grafts, groin

Informed consent

Before any procedure the patient must give an informed consent for the surgery. For full informed consent you should discuss:

- what the procedure involves
- alternatives to the procedure
- common risks, e.g. pain, bruising, scar, time to heal
- risks with consequences, e.g. infections
- site-specific considerations, e.g. ectropion
- patient expectations

You should also mention lifestyle adjustments that will facilitate wound healing. Give the patient written information about common risks and postoperative care.

Postoperative patient information should include advice:

- to avoid alcohol on the day of procedure
- to limit strenuous activity for 2 weeks

- not to stretch at the site for 4 weeks
- to use sunscreen on the wound for 3 months
- to sleep with head elevated (facial surgery)

18.5 Suturing

Sutures are either absorbable or non-absorbable (superficial sutures) and made from a variety of materials (**Table 18.3**). The size of the suture is based on its tensile strength and not diameter. Different suture sizes are best used at certain body sites (**Table 18.4**).

Technique

Wound eversion is the key to optimal wound healing. The wound margin should be an elevated ridge above the surrounding skin with the two dermal edges in full contact with each other (**Figure 18.7**).

Superficial sutures
Simple interrupted suture (Figure 18.8)
Step 1 Insert the needle tip at 90° to the skin so the semicircular needle is arched over the skin surface.
Step 2 Guide the needle through the skin in an arc by rotating the wrist, exiting the epidermis on the opposite side of the wound – the stitch should be slightly wider at its deep aspect.
Step 3 Tie the suture: on the first pass wind the long end of the suture around the needle holder twice and pull the free end through to lie flat on the wound. On the second pass wrap the long end around in the reverse direction once, and pull the short end through so that it lies flat on the first tie and makes a square knot. Repeat this for a third pass.
Step 4 Cut the suture 4–5 mm above the knot.

Vertical mattress suture (Figure 18.9)
Step 1 Perform a simple interrupted suture, without tying it.
Step 2 Turn the needle in the opposite direction and re-enter the epidermis, this time 2–4 mm further away from the wound margin, passing the needle through the subcutaneous tissue

	Type	Memory	Tissue reactivity	Tensile strength half-life	Uses
Non-absorbable					
Ethilon, Monosof (nylon)	Monofilament	High	Low	–	Skin surface
Prolene (polypropylene)	Monofilament	Very high	Very low	–	Skin surface, running subcuticular
Silk	Braided/twisted	Very low	High	–	Mucosa
Absorbable					
Chromic catgut	Twisted	Very high	High	1 week	Mucosa; grafts
Vicryl/Polysorb (polyglactin 910)	Braided	Very low	Low	2 weeks	Subcutaneous closure, vessel ligation
Monocryl (poliglecaprone 25)	Monofilament	Low	Very low	1 week	Subcutaneous closure (low reactivity)
Maxon (polyglyconate)	Monofilament	Low	Very low	1 month	Subcutaneous closure (high tension)
PDS (polydoxanone)	Monofilament	High	Very low	1 month	Subcutaneous closure (high tension)

Table 18.3 Suture material

Body site	Timing of suture removal (days)	Common suture (USP) used
Lower limb	14	3/0, 4/0
Trunk/abdomen	10	3/0, 4/0
Upper limb	7	4/0
Head and neck	5–7	4/0 or 5/0 (subcuticular), 5/0 or 6/0 (surface)
Genitals/mucosae	Use absorbable sutures	4/0 or 5/0
USP, United States Pharmacopeia.		

Table 18.4 Suture suggestions for different body site

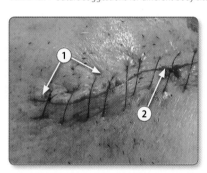

Figure 18.7 Wound eversion. ① Good eversion and alignment. ② Slight misalignment on the superior border.

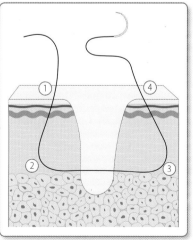

Figure 18.8 Simple interrupted suture. 1–4 represent the order the needle should pass through the skin.

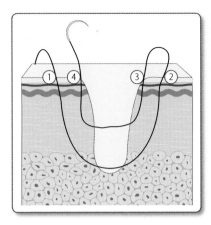

Figure 18.9 Vertical mattress suture. 1–4 represent the order the needle should pass through the skin.

(deeper than the first pass), surfacing 2–4 mm on the far side of the original entry point. The entry–exit points are near–near then far–far.

Step 3 Tie off the suture.

Deep sutures

Subcutaneous interrupted suture (Figure 18.10)

These are vital to obtain a low tension for epidermal wound closure for low-tension wound closure.

Step 1 After undermining, pass the needle from the deep surface of the subcutaneous tissue/fat and push it inwards towards the wound margin, exiting the mid-/deep dermis.

Step 2 Enter the mid-/deep dermis (the same level as finishing step 1) on the other side of the wound and push the needle into the subcutaneous tissue to match the placement in step 1.

Step 3 Tie off the suture; cut the suture at the level of the knot, burying it.

18.6 Postoperative care and dressings

Application of an occlusive dressing over an acute wound results in 40% more rapid healing due to the moist environment.

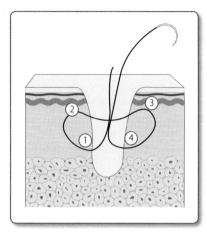

Figure 18.10 Deep sutures. 1–4 represent the order the needle should pass through the skin.

The ideal dressing:
- enhances epithelial migration
- stimulates angiogenesis, deposition of collagen
- allows retention of growth factors
- protects from exogenous organisms
- absorbs excess exudate

Common complications that patients may encounter after surgery include:
- bruising – apply ice for <20 min
- scar – massage, topical silicone, intralesional triamcinolone
- infection – swab and start empirical oral antibiotics
- haematoma – sutures should be removed and the haematoma aspirated

18.7 Surgical procedures

Diagnostic skin biopsies must be taken from a representative lesion or part of the rash. For tumours or larger lesions, this is best taken from the edge of the lesion, including a small margin of normal skin for comparison. For therapeutic procedures the entire lesion should be removed with a margin of clinically normal skin.

The various methods of obtaining skin for histology are outlined below.

Shave biopsy

Antiseptic is used to clean the site. The lesion is slowly injected intradermally with LA to elevate it from the surrounding skin. A scalpel blade is used to slice the specimen from the skin at the level of the superficial dermis (**Figure 18.11**). After electrocautery the remaining defect is a shallow disc that will heal by secondary intention as a flat or slightly depressed hypopigmented scar.

Saucerisation

This is similar to a shave but is performed to a greater dermal depth to increase tumour clearance.

Curettage

A curette (range in size: 3–7 mm) is used to remove the tumour by passing it from the central tumour to the periphery of the tumour in a scraping motion (**Figure 18.12**). In this way balls

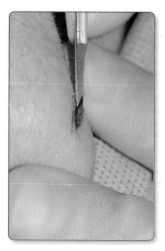

Figure 18.11 Shave biopsy.

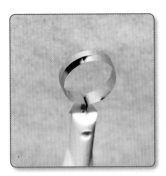

Figure 18.12 Curettage.

or strips of tissue are removed, because the tumour tissue is more friable than normal skin. One or two further passes can also be done after electrocautery to remove residual disease.

Punch biopsy

A punch biopsy is taken with a punch tool 2–8 mm in diameter (usually 4 mm). After LA, and antiseptic wash, the skin is stretched perpendicular to the RSTL and the tool is held at 90° to the skin. It is rotated (in one direction, to avoid epidermal shearing), cutting through the epidermis and dermis, and into the subcutaneous fat (**Figure 18.13**). The specimen is cut free at the base if necessary. This produces a round column of skin for histology and an elliptical defect, closed by inserting one or two cutaneous sutures.

Elliptical excision

The following steps should be followed when performing an elliptical excision of a lesion:

- The lesion to be excised is marked out with an adequate margin.
- An ellipse is drawn to encompass the outer margin. The long axis is oriented along the RSTL so that it is approximately three times as long as it is wide (**Figure 18.14**).
- LA is infiltrated.
- The skin is prepared with antiseptic using an aseptic technique.

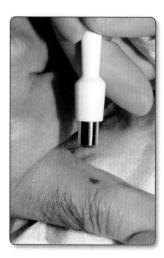

Figure 18.13 An excisional punch biopsy.

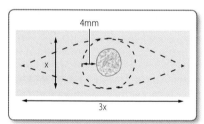

Figure 18.14 Elliptical excision illustating the margin required to excise a nodular basal cell carcinoma.

- Holding the scalpel perpendicularly, score the skin along the marking, then cut to the level of the subcutaneous fat with the scalpel belly.
- Bluntly dissect and remove the entire ellipse.
- Undermine about 1–2 cm lateral to wound edge with blunt dissection.
- Electrocauterise any bleeding points.
- Insert enough subcutaneous interrupted sutures to appose and elevate the wound edges.

Superficial cutaneous interrupted sutures are then placed.

Destructive methods

Cryotherapy can be used to treat skin tumours or premalignant lesions, but there is no tissue for histology confirmation, so cryotherapy should be performed where the diagnosis is certain. It is useful for:

- actinic keratoses
- viral warts
- seborrhoeic keratoses and other benign lesions
- low-risk basal cell carcinomas (BCCs)
- Bowen's disease

Clinical insight

Blunt dissection is performed by inserting scissors horizontally into the fat plane, opening them, inserting again just laterally and repeating, snipping the tissue strands between the passes.

Laser surgery is discussed further in section 18.10 (page 303).

18.8 Skin cancer surgical procedures

Wide local excision

Benign tumours require a smaller excision margin than malignant lesions (**Table 18.5**). Tissue shrinks around 20% during histological processing and this should be taken into account when marking clinical margins before excision.

Mohs' micrographic surgery

The process of Mohs' micrographic excisions is outlined in Figure 18.15. It differs from standard excision in the following ways.

- The surgical excision margin is examined in its entirety (100% of the peripheral and deep margin is seen) as a flattened disc
- It is tissue conserving, minimising the rim of normal tissue excised
- Surgical margin clearance is obtained before reconstruction
- It offers higher cure rate for contiguous tumours

It is the gold standard for treatment of some skin cancers but is usually reserved for the following situations.

- **High-risk BCC:** sites of high recurrence (periocular, nose, lips, ears), tumours >2 cm, high-risk subtypes (morphoeic, infiltrative, micronodular, basosquamous), recurrent lesions, poorly defined, perineural or perivascular involvement
- **High-risk squamous cell carcinoma (SCC):** those on the

Tumour	Clinical excision margins (mm)	Recommended histological margin (mm)
Benign lesion (e.g. dermatofibroma)	1–2	Minimal
Basal cell carcinoma	4–5	>3
Squamous cell carcinoma	4–5 (6 if high risk)	>4
Benign naevus	2–3	>1
Melanoma in situ	>5	>5
Tumour	**Breslow's thickness (mm)**	**Margin (mm) of wide local excision**
Malignant melanoma (dependent on tumour thickness)	<1 1–2 >2	10 10–20 20

Table 18.5 Recommended excision margins for different lesions

lip/ear/perineum, sole of foot, >2 cm, high-risk subtype, perineural invasion, recurrent tumours
- **high-risk patients:** immunosuppressed patients and those with Gorlin's syndrome or xeroderma pigmentosum

Mohs' surgery is used to treat lentigo maligna, dermatofibrosarcoma protuberans, sebaceous carcinomas, microcystic adnexal carcinoma, Merkel's cell carcinoma, Paget's disease of the breast and sarcoma.

18.9 Reconstruction

After tumour removal by Mohs' micrographic surgery or wide excision (low-risk lesions), the defect must be repaired. A number of factors influence this decision, which can be divided into:
- patient factors:
  - patient preference, cosmetic concerns, frailty
  - comorbidities: diabetes, hypertension, peripheral vascular disease
  - smoking history
- defect factors:

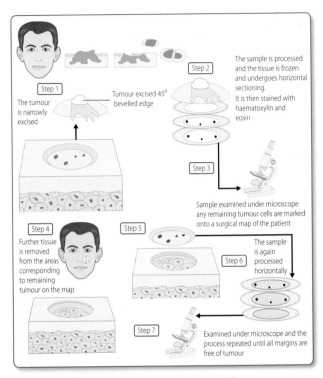

Figure 18.15 Mohs' micrographic surgery.

- – size, shape and depth
- – surrounding skin laxity – tissue reserve
- – RSTL and cosmetic subunits
- – anatomical function

The reconstructive ladder

This describes the order in which reconstructive procedures are considered, from simple to more complex approaches (**Table 18.6**).

Secondary intention healing
Primary closure – may be linear, curvilinear
Local flaps – advancement, rotation, transposition
Full-thickness skin graft
Distant skin flaps

Table 18.6 The reconstructive ladder

Secondary intention healing

This is the simplest level on the reconstructive ladder. Time to complete wound healing depends on the size of the defect's area. It requires regular cleaning and simple, moist, non-adherent, occlusive wound dressings.

This method is suitable for some concave surfaces (ear concha, pre-/postauricular areas) and occasionally the dorsum of the hand and lower legs.

Linear side-to-side closure

Undermining can enable a linear closure if there is no pull on adjacent free margins and minimal wound tension (**Figure 18.16**).

Consider the technique for small defects and older patients with lax skin.

Advancement flaps These involve displacing Burow's triangle to a more convenient location (**Figure 18.17**). Tissue movement occurs in a straight line. The length:width should be <3:1.

Consider the technique for forehead, hairline, perialar region (crescentic – **Figure 18.18**) and above/below the eye.

Rotation flaps These are constructed by converting the defect into a triangle and taking a long curved (usually the length is 4 times that of the defect width) incision from the defect edge around the tissue reservoir (**Figure 18.19**). Insertion of a back cut into the pedicle of the flap can enhance flap mobility. The tissue is rotated in a fan shape.

Consider for cheek, temple or scalp/forehead.

Transposition flaps These involve reorientation from an adjacent donor site that has greater skin laxity (**Figure 18.20**).

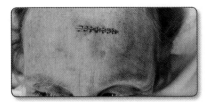

Figure 18.16 Linear side-to-side closure.

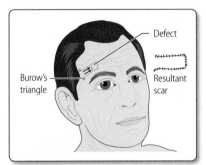

Figure 18.17 Advancement flap.

Defect

Burow's triangle

Resultant scar

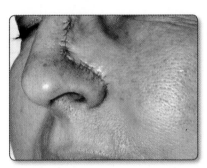

Figure 18.18 Perialar advancement flap.

It allows for redirection of the tension to avoid pull on the free margins. The flap is incised, undermined and then pivoted on a pedicle to transpose it over the defect. The donor site is closed first and primarily, and the flap trimmed to match the defect shape.

Consider for nose tip/side wall (bilobed, nasolabial fold flap), temple, cheek and chin.

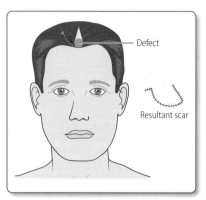

Figure 18.19 Rotation flap.

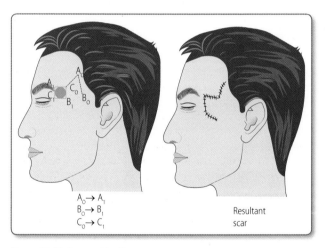

Figure 18.20 Transposition flap.

Skin grafts

A graft may be:
- split thickness of the skin
- full thickness of the skin
- composite – skin and cartilage

Donor sites include upper eyelid, pre-/postauricular area, supraclavicular fossa and conchal bowl, and should be matched to the defect site colour and texture.

Consider for nasal tip, ala, sidewall, lower eyelid and ear; consider composite grafts for deep nasal alar defect, eyelids and helix.

Distant flaps

This is when a flap of skin is raised from a site distant to the defect and is sutured to the recipient wound bed to the defect by means of a connecting 'bridge', (or pedicle) allowing the blood supply at the recipient site to develop. The bridge of skin is divided 3 weeks later. Consider for full-thickness nasal defects and eyelid margin defects.

18.10 Laser surgery

Background

Lasers (laser = light amplification by stimulated emission of radiation) are a useful treatment adjunct in dermatological surgery. They may be used to cut, coagulate or ablate tissue, and also to treat a wide range of skin conditions including hyperpigmentation (e.g. melasma), cutaneous vascular lesions (e.g. haemangiomas), telangiectasias (e.g. in rosacea) and small varicose veins, unwanted hair removal and skin resurfacing/rejuvenation. They are also used to remove tattoos. There are many different types of lasers and their properties (e.g. wavelength, energy) determine which type of skin lesion they are most suitable to treat. The aim of laser treatment is to destroy the target cells (e.g. small vessels in port wine stains) without injuring adjacent normal cells.

Principles and terminology

The basic principle of medical lasers is the emission of photons of electromagnetic energy, also known as high-intensity light. The light is monochromatic (photons are of a single wavelength), coherent (light beam waves are in phase) and collimated (the beams travel in parallel).

The light is produced in a laser medium. The medium may be gas (e.g. carbon dioxide), liquid (e.g. dye) or solid (e.g. ruby). An energy source (usually electrical current running through the laser medium) is used to excite electrons in molecules/atoms of the laser medium from the ground state to a higher energy level. The electrons then quickly return to their ground state from the excited state and emit coherent photons of light of a characteristic wavelength.

The clinical utility of lasers is governed by the following:

- Laser wavelength: the longer the wavelength of the laser, the greater the depth of penetration in the skin. Longer-wavelength lasers penetrate into the dermis and may be used for deeper skin lesions.
- Chromophores: these are the molecules absorbing the energy, e.g. melanin and haemoglobin.

The wavelength of the photon determines the depth to which it is absorbed in the skin and by which chromophore in the skin. Only a laser that has a wavelength absorbed by melanin is suitable for treating pigmented lesions.

Pulse duration

The duration of the laser pulse is determined by the thermal relaxation time of the chromophore. Thermal relaxation time is the time required for the tissue temperature to return to its baseline temperature. If a target is heated for longer than its thermal relaxation time, the surrounding tissue can be damaged.

The following terms should be understood when discussing lasers:

- energy: defined as the capacity to do work and measured in joules
- power: the rate of doing work, measured in watts (joules/s)
- fluence: this is the energy delivered per unit area measured in joules/cm^2
- irradiance: the power per unit area measured in watts/cm^2

Lasers commonly used in dermatology are shown in **Table 18.7**.

Laser	Wavelength (nm)	Indications
Pulsed dye laser	585–595	Vascular malformations Hypertrophic scar
Nd:YAG	1064	Deep pigment, telangiectasia
Q-switch Nd:Yag	1064, 532	Tattoo, pigmentation
Alexandrite	755	Epilation
CO_2	10 600	Resurfacing, scarring
Nd:YAG, neodymium:yttrium–aluminium–garnet.		

Table 18.7 Lasers in dermatology

18.11 Cosmetic dermatology

Cosmetic dermatology is a rapidly growing area within dermatology. It is important to understand the procedures and potential complications, and how to deal with them. Patient consent, expectations, selection and psychological assessment are of the utmost importance.

Resurfacing procedures injure the skin in a controlled manner to stimulate growth of new skin. It can be done via chemical (peel) or physical (laser) methods. The deeper the resurfacing, the greater the effect, but there are increased risks of complications.

Chemical peels are performed for actinic damage, scarring or pigment disorders. Before a peel, cleansing is performed with acetone to remove debris. A test spot is usually performed at the hairline. The peel solution is applied until erythema, in some cases frosting, is evident. Clinical experience is required to determine the appropriate end-point (**Table 18.8**).

Complications

The complications are:
- infections: *Staphylococcus aureus*/herpes simplex virus (HSV)

Depth	Physical ablation methods	Type of peel
Very superficial (epidermis exfoliation)	Microdermabrasion	α-Hydroxy acids (glycolic acid) 10–20% trichloroacetic acid (TCA) Topical tretinoin 20% salicylic acid (melasma) Jessner's solution (4% resorcinol, 14% lactic and 14% salicylic acid in alcohol)
Superficial (epidermis/ superficial papillary dermis)	Microdermabrasion	50–70% glycolic acid Jessner's solution 25–30% TCA 30% salicylic acid
Medium depth (papillary/upper reticular dermis)	Manual dermasanding Er:YAG laser Superficial CO_2 laser	Jessner's solution–30% TCA 70% glycolic acid–35% TCA
Deep (mid-reticular dermis)	Manual dermasanding CO_2 laser	Baker's phenol croton oil – not recommended
Er:YAG, erbium:yttrium–aluminium–garnet.		

Table 18.8 Chemical peels

- hyper- /hypopigmentation: increased risk with skin types IV–VI
- textural irregularity
- prolonged erythema
- scarring

Botulinum toxin (BTX) This exists as several strains (A–G) derived from *Clostridium botulinum*. BTX blocks release of acetylcholine from the presynaptic nerve terminal and paralyses the muscles of facial expression that cause dynamic (movement-associated) wrinkles. The toxin also denervates the eccrine glands and is useful for hyperhidrosis. The effect lasts 3–6 months. Different formulations, such as onabotulinum toxin A (Botox) and abobotulinum toxin A (Dysport), are not interchangeable for units or dosage.

Common injection sites are:

- glabella (muscles targeted are procerus and corrugator supercilli)
- lateral to orbital margin ('crows' feet' – the muscle targeted is orbicularis oculi)
- horizontal forehead (muscle targeted is frontalis)
- lateral sides of root of the nose ('bunny lines' – muscle targeted is nasalis)
- hyperhidrosis on the axilla, palms and soles which can be treated with BTX

Complications of treatment include bruising, ptosis, antibody formation (BTX becomes ineffective) and allergy (very rare).

Soft-tissue augmentation This can be used to 'plump' or fill facial soft tissue hollows associated with disease or ageing or to ameliorate wrinkles in areas such as nasolabial folds, vertical lip wrinkles or marionette lines. **Table 18.9** outlines the different sources of augmentation material and the associated complications.

Category/ composition	Proprietary name	Use	Duration (months)	Complications
Autologous fat transfer	NA	Large areas of volume loss	May be permanent	Requires harvesting liposuction, incision, pain, bleeding
Bovine collagen	Zyderm I/II Zyplast (glutaraldehyde linked – less immunogenic)	Wrinkles (superficial dermis), lips	2–4	3% incidence of allergy – double skin testing required at 0, 2 weeks; granuloma, over-correction required

Table 18.9 *Continued...*

Category/ composition	Proprietary name	Use	Duration (months)	Complications
Hyaluronic acid	Restylane Fine Lines (smaller particles)	Wrinkles (superficial dermis), perioral lines	4–6	Painful injection without lidocaine, papules/ nodules/ granulomas, 0.4% risk of allergy
	Restylane	Wrinkles (mid-dermis), lips	6–12	
	Perlane – larger particle	Deeper wrinkles (deep dermis)	6–12	
	Hylaform/ HylanB	Wrinkles, lips	3–4	
Human collagen	Cosmoderm	Wrinkles, superficial dermis	2–4	
	Cosmoplast	Deeper wrinkles		
Poly-l-lactic acid	Sculptra	Volume loss in HIV, nasolabial folds/deeper wrinkles (superficial sub-cutaneous fat)	>1 year	Non-visible papule formation

Table 18.9 Soft-tissue augmentation materials

Index

Note: Page numbers in **bold** or *italic* refer to tables or figures respectively.

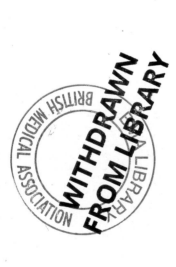